Experiments in Love and Death

Experiments in Love and Death
Medicine, Postmodernism, Microethics and the Body

Paul A Komesaroff

MONASH UNIVERSITY, MELBOURNE, AUSTRALIA
DIRECTOR, CENTRE FOR THE STUDY OF ETHICS IN
MEDICINE AND SOCIETY

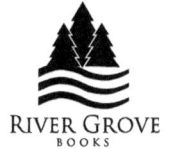

RIVER GROVE
BOOKS

Published by River Grove Books
Austin, TX
www.rivergrovebooks.com

Copyright ©2008 Paul A. Komesaroff

All rights reserved.

No part of this book may be reproduced, stored in a retrieval system, or transmitted by any means, electronic, mechanical, photocopying, recording, or otherwise, without written permission from the copyright holder.

Distributed by River Grove Books

For ordering information or special discounts for bulk purchases, please contact River Grove Books at PO Box 91869, Austin, TX 78709, 512.891.6100.

Design by Phil Campbell
Previously published by Melbourne University Press, an imprint of Melbourne University Publishing Limited.

Publisher's Cataloging-In-Publication Data

Komesaroff, Paul A.
  Experiments in love and death : medicine, postmodernism, microethics, and the body / Paul A. Komesaroff, Director, Monash Centre for the Study of Ethics in Medicine and Society, Monash University, Melbourne, Australia.—First edition.

  pages ; cm

  Previously published: Melbourne University Press, 2008.
  Issued also as an ebook.
  Includes bibliographical references and index.
  ISBN: 978-1-938416-97-2

  1. Medical ethics. 2. Medicine—Decision making—Moral and ethical aspects. 3. Physician and patient—Moral and ethical aspects. 4. Postmodernism. I. Title.

R724 .K66 2014
174.2   2014937210
Komesaroff, Paul A.

Print ISBN: 978-1-938416-97-2

First Edition

For Sally, Frida and Ilya

Contents

Acknowledgements		viii
Foreword by Alphonso Lingis		ix
The Practice of Ethics: A Manifesto		xiii

Part I: Medicine, Postmodernism, Microethics and the Body

1.	Medicine and the Ethical Conditions of Modernity	3
2.	From Bioethics to Microethics: The Need to Return Ethical Debate to the Clinic	20
3.	Between Nature and Culture: The Ethics and Politics of Animal Experimentation	47
4.	Sexuality and Ethics in the Medical Encounter	72
5.	The Medicalisation of Everyday Life and the Moral Space of the Menopausal Woman	101

Part II: Love and Death

6.	The Many Faces of the Clinic	123
7.	The Experience of Evil	139
8.	Death Sentence	157
9.	Time, Ethics and the Archive	177
10.	At the Gates of the Labyrinth	192
11.	How to End a Life	211
12.	Fardels of the Heart	226
13.	The Case of Miss T	246

Epilogue	265
Index	271

Acknowledgements

The essays in this book draw on the experiences of many people whom I have come to know through my professional work. Where possible, I have obtained permission from them to refer to their cases, subject, of course, to changing factual details to protect confidentiality. I would like to express my deep appreciation to these people for the privilege of being able to talk with and to serve them, and to learn from their courage, wisdom and generosity.

Permission to quote from previous versions of the following chapters is gratefully acknowledged:

Chapter 1, from 'The Ethical Conditions of Modernity', in J Daly, ed., *Ethical Intersections* (Sydney, Allen and Unwin, 1996).

Chapter 2, from 'From Bioethics to Microethics: The Need to Return Bioethics to the Clinic', in PA Komesaroff, ed., *Troubled Bodies* (Durham, Duke University Press, and Melbourne, Melbourne University Press, 1995).

Chapter 3 from 'Nature and Culture: The Case of Animal Experimentation', in *Thesis 11*, 32, June 1992: 55–75.

Chapter 5, from 'The Moral Space of the Menopausal Woman', in PA Komesaroff, P Rothfield and J Daly, eds, *Reinterpreting Menopause: Philosophical and Ethical Issues* (United States, Routledge, 1997), pp. 54–74.

Chapter 6, from 'The Many Faces of the Clinic: A Levinasian View', in SK Toombs, ed., *Handbook for the Philosophy of Medicine, Volume One: Phenomenology and Medicine* (Dordrecht, The Netherlands, Kluwer Academic Publishers, 2001), pp. 317–30.

Chapter 13, from 'The Case of Miss T.', in H Kuhse, ed., *Willing to Listen, Wanting to Die* (Melbourne, Penguin, 1994).

I thank the many friends, colleagues and students who have supported, sustained and enriched me over the years through inspiration, ideas, and the 'miracle of conversation'. I would like especially to express my gratitude to my family, including my mother Dessa and late father Moische, my sisters Ilona and Ruth, and above all, my partner Sally and children Frida and Ilya, from whom I have learnt the most.

Foreword

This important book situates ethics in medical practice in a radically new way. Ethics, which aims to establish values and principles for action, has been set up as a discourse of a different kind from the empirical discourse of medical science. Ethical judgements are perceived to be outside interventions in the autonomous progression of medical science and practice. Political and economic discourse and practice are likewise external to the discourse of medical science, and ethical considerations are seen to be imposed from the outside upon the political and economic discussions that determine the funding of medical care. The discourse of cultural and religious values and prohibitions are external to the discourse of medical science.

Dr Paul Komesaroff analyses the clinical experience. A patient comes to the doctor for the diagnosis and treatment of illness or suspected illness, for advice about avoiding medical problems, for assistance with the passage through natural processes like pregnancy and menopause, or for help in dealing with marital or social problems that follow illness or death. The patient submits his or her body to medical scrutiny, but that body is not only a biochemical organism. It is also a body traumatised or empowered with past afflictions; a body whose powers are channelled into specific kinds of actions, functioning with rational, symbolic, cultural and perhaps religious meanings; a body whose functioning is coordinated and conflicted with the bodies of others; a body with sexual drives and aesthetic preoccupations with itself; a body whose functioning is constrained or empowered with material resources and sociopolitical forces. The doctor must diagnose the medical problem not only with laboratory tests, but also with the patient's account of the origins and symptoms of the distress. The patient speaks often with learned scientifico-medical terminology but also in colloquial language, language specific to age or ethnic groups, sometimes conveying social prejudice or political outlook. The doctor's speech is not simply a citation of relevant passages of medical science and reports of laboratory tests, but also greets, signifies listening, invites further elucidation, interprets, confirms, enjoins behaviours, provokes, persuades and also voices baleful prognoses, confronts the patient with the limits where despair, but also the possibility of insight and wisdom, are possible.

The doctor is there not only as a voice, but also speaks with his or her physical presence and hands. The doctor must make decisions with family members of the patient.

Dr Komesaroff finds that the clinical interaction is intrinsically ethical. The doctor maintains responsibility for the patient's biological body, shaped by past traumas and by present commitments to work and to social, political and economic possibilities and constraints. The patient does not live without maintaining responsibility for his or her activities, engagements with work and with others, his or her state of wellbeing, illness and oncoming death. The clinical experience involves mistakes, accidents and unpredictable consequences of treatments. Ethical consciousness and decision-making require communication between these multiple and divergent responsibilities, which form an individual configuration in each clinical interaction.

It is not a matter of treating the 'whole' patient. The doctor has access to no more than a fragment of the patient's life—that part for which he or she has come to the clinic for attention. Nor is it a matter of adding empathy and friendship to the clinical discourse, as these may well hinder critical reflection on the part of both doctor and patient.

Dr Komesaroff sets out to clarify the nature of this ethical reflection and the kind of discourse with which it is formulated. This ethical discourse cannot be formulated in universal categories and juridical reasonings. It is not concerned with truth but with validity. It is not a discourse about good but rather about the avoidance of evil, and even about the positive use of evil to determine the limits of meaning. Dr Komesaroff calls it microethics.

He explains how microethical reflection came to be passed over as biomedical ethics was set up as an autonomous discourse, exterior to the language of medical science. With economy, precision and clarity, he explains how, nonetheless, biomedical ethics and medical science—as well as psychological, sociological, political and economic discourses that likewise were set up as autonomous discourses—share fundamental assumptions as to the nature of reason, evidence and argument. Ethical value was given to the promotion of this kind of reason. These fundamental assumptions have paradoxically made these discourses exterior to one another, and exterior to the kind of reflection and decision-making that occur within the clinical encounter. The fundamental assumptions they share that make proponents and opponents of animal experimentation in medical research unable to resolve issues, because they are unable to communicate, is a case in point.

Reading this book convinces us that the public discussions of professional ethicists and jurists, when they have made their decisions and inscribed their legislation, will not have resolved the ethical decisions that doctors and also patients have to make. To be theoretically sound and practically useful, these decisions will have to arise out of the practice of microethics. This insight has far-reaching consequences for theorists of ethics in every domain. Do we not need a microethics for research ethics, environmental ethics and teaching ethics? We are aware of concrete cases where legal ethics, journalist ethics and, indeed, government ethics and business ethics are not settled by establishing professional codes of conduct. Do we not need microethics in these areas also?

Medical science does not simply result from experimentation, but, given the complexity and singularity of every patient's full body, medical practice will be some kind of experimentation. And the practice of ethical responsibility within the clinical encounter will also be an experimentation. Ethical decisions will issue from an experimentation by the patient—and by the doctor—with ways of suffering, healing and dying. Dr Komesaroff examines cases where ethical reflection turns out to be groping and progressive and an experimentation with love and death: a woman whose present medical problems in menopause are tied to deep and incurable psychic wounds; a woman whose ovaries and uterus were wrongly surgically removed, and who is now prostrate with incapacitating pain; a woman orphaned as a child in Auschwitz and now suffering an incapacitating menopause; people facing incurable medical conditions; an athletic woman stricken with multiple sclerosis; a woman blocked in obesity; a woman for whom both scientific and alternative treatments for cancer have failed; a man awaiting a donor heart for transplant, kept alive with an LVAD machine after the transplant becomes medically impossible; caregivers and family whose lives become nothing but suffering. In these clinical encounters, where biomedical ethics falter and fail, Dr Komesaroff shows what microethical reflection is at work, and how it does not revert to relativism or subjectivism but guides responsibility and action.

Out of microethical reflection in these singular cases, Dr Komesaroff develops far-reaching insights with subtle care. His experience illuminates what suffering is: it does not in itself have meaning but can generate meanings. Suffering is not a property of the individual sufferer; it is from the first shared and exists between individuals. He sees the clash of two forms of inevitable incomprehension before suffering: that of the afflicted patient and that of the institutional structures of medical practice. He discovers how clinical medicine opens access to the most intimate recesses of that person's being, challenging meanings, undermining assumptions and provoking fundamental reassessments and revaluations. For the clinical relationship is not just one of support and affirmation, but also of subversion and confrontation. He confronts the problem of understanding a patient's will to undergo certain treatments or to be allowed to die when that will was expressed in earlier and different circumstances and when it can no longer express itself. He reflects on evil—on what it is like to be a victim of unjust or cruel behaviour— and finds that the experience of having been a victim of evil can play a constructive and affirmative role in the stabilisation of meaning and values for all of us.

He sees that the doctor is not only agent but witness, and explores the meaning of that witness. Whether the medical intervention cures, sustains palliatively or fails, the doctor is there to record, constitute an active memory, organise experiences and render them intelligible, and define possibilities for the future. He is there as a witness to the lives and sufferings of patients whose lives and sufferings are perhaps otherwise unknown and uncommemorated.

This is an essential book for doctors, nurses and caregivers. It is also a book for all of us, destined to suffer and to die, and responsible in our suffering and death—responsible for ourselves and for our loved ones and comrades. And it is written with a clarity, discretion and sensitivity that will hold the attention of every reader. Anyone who reads this book will keep it to be re-read in days of distress ahead and to share it with friends.

Alphonso Lingis
Baltimore, MD
March 2008

The Practice of Ethics: A Manifesto

This book is concerned with how to think about and practise ethics. It takes as its point of departure a paradox at the heart of contemporary ethical experience.

Ethics is called upon simultaneously to serve two very different tasks. On the one hand, it poses difficult questions about underlying assumptions, values and goals, reasons and justifications to help guide decisions and actions. This function of ethics is radical and inexorably subversive. It takes nothing for granted and respects no authority. On the other hand, ethics is at the same time called upon to serve an opposite function—to regulate conduct and to ensure that all social actors do what is accepted of them, that they act in a prudent and predictable way. In this function, there is no room for radical questioning or risky iconoclasm. If society is to function smoothly, there is a need for stable, predicable patters of behaviour, and this is what ethics seeks to deliver.

The paradox is reflected in the discussions and debates about ethics that proliferate in the academic and popular literature. In fact, in recent years there has been an explosion of interest in ethics, especially in the fields of medicine and science where it is widely acknowledged that perplexing ethical issues abound. The popular media, clinical practitioners, journals and institutional committees all engage in vigorous, sometimes furious, arguments about ethics, and teaching programs in medicine, nursing and related disciplines now invariably include material on ethical decision-making.[1]

The increased interest in ethics, however, is not restricted to clinical medicine but includes many other fields too. We also have research ethics, environmental ethics, business ethics, science ethics, legal ethics, teaching ethics, military ethics, journalist ethics, computer ethics, government ethics, sporting ethics, accountancy ethics and many more. In all these fields, 'experts' commonly offer their opinions on key questions to provide answers to dilemmas, large and small. We can read in the newspaper about whether we are ethically obliged to vote in elections, whether we should stop at red lights, ask people their occupations, open doors for others, or how we should end a love affair or respond to a drunk in the street. There is much public discussion about whether one should be a vegetarian, wear clothes made of fur, use air conditioning, drive a car or give money to charity.

There are several likely reasons for the increased interest in ethics. For many, modern life is experienced as darkly threatening and precipitous, and the task of finding meaning and making decisions about personal conduct is daunting and oppressive; for others, the expanding possibilities open up new, rich opportunities for reflection and change. It is possible that the enhanced profile of ethics reflects an increased sense of uncertainty about how to act in a world of growing complexity, a desire to find answers to increasingly difficult questions about technology and the proliferation of cultures and value systems. It may reflect greater awareness of the range of moral choice in an era of increased communication and globalised economic and political discourses.

My focus in this book is on the ethical issues arising within medicine, primarily within Western, developed societies, although many of the considerations apply increasingly to the globalised cultures of so-called 'developing' societies. The ethical issues occur at many levels. They occur in relation to large-scale questions about values and society, about our relationships with each other and with nature, about the impact of new developments in science and medical treatments, and the extent to which we should embrace these innovations or take steps to contain them. They occur in relation to the nature of the social relationships, the so-called 'regional' relationships of trust and power, which can be both the source of confidence and caring and of exploitation and betrayal. And they occur at the level of individual experience, the local or 'microethical' level, where one person engages another face to face, where we encounter suffering and pain, bitterness and gratitude, love and resentment, caring and trust.

In individual cases many issues may come together. To quote a personal example, I might be faced with the dilemma of whether or how I should care for my ageing mother who is suffering from severe memory loss that has been diagnosed as Alzheimer's disease.[2] I may consider questions of a personal nature in relation to society generally and perhaps to wider philosophical and social considerations. I may reflect on my personal relationship with her, the debt that I owe her for the love and care she has provided to me, and on questions about the distribution of resources in a society that is itself ageing. I may wonder about my personal responsibilities and the responsibilities of society in general to care for its older citizens. In practice, I may encounter all these issues within the flux of my everyday life, in the context of my other relationships and activities.

******

Although my primary concern in this book is with medicine, many of the discussions within it are of wider relevance. Ethical considerations inhabit the very core of our sense of who we are. They reflect the primordial, irrefragable bond we have with others that is the condition of all meaning and value. They arise out of the responsibility we unavoidably incur simply as a condition of being human. These experiences of ethics include, but are not restricted to, the purely cognitive or philosophical: we do not come to ethical decisions purely through a process of thinking or rational argument. We draw on the whole range and variety of our embodied, sensuous lives, our memories of illness and pain, sexuality and love, and our hopes and fears about the future.[3]

To recognise that ethics plays a fundamental role in our lives does not, of course, tell us how to act. Decisions about what we should do may remain difficult despite our enhanced ethical sensitivity. This may be because the circumstances with which we are dealing are uncertain and complex or because we ourselves may feel ambivalence or conflicting emotions. Sometimes the facts have multiple interpretations or there are intractably opposed forces at play. It is a common discovery, for example, that illness, pain and physical suffering can become fecund sources of insight and wisdom, and may greatly deepen relationships and engender new purposes and hope. Or things can go the other way. Advancing technologies can bring major benefits, including pleasure, the relief of illness, or access to new possibilities; however, by displacing activities with ethical content in favour of purely technical ones, they can also lead to an erosion of meaning, to a degradation of intimate human experiences and the undermining of traditional, community-based systems of meaning generation.[4]

Ethical theory has been created to help with sorting through this uncertainty and complexity. For all its popularity, however, the gains have been much less than they seem. This is partly because of the paradox mentioned at the start of this chapter: while ethical thought can facilitate and provoke fundamental questioning, at the same time it also tends to impose limits on what is possible, to ensure conformity to existing social norms or patterns of thought. In fact, the conservatism has usually predominated, even among ethical theories presented by their authors as radical and iconoclastic. For all the sound and the fury, the dominant ethical discourses have not in general supported a deep questioning of the conditions and assumptions that generated the problems they are seeking to solve. This in turn reflects the fact that the inexorable forces driving modern society forward—including science and medicine, money and power—also sweep up ethical discourse, which is therefore implicated within and co-opted by it.

Theories of Ethics in the Modern Age

Ethical theory is certainly not monolithic. It draws on a range of traditions and incorporates a wide range of theoretical perspectives; for example, within the Western tradition, Aristotelianism, deontology, utilitarianism, neo-Aristotelianism, 'principlism', egoism, narrative theory, discourse theory, relativism and feminist ethics, to name just a few. Many of these theoretical approaches propose ways of generating normative rules and of solving 'dilemmas'. As may be expected, each has its limitations, and all have been subjected to detailed, critical scrutiny. For example, bioethics, itself a cluster of theories that has been among the most influential of the contemporary approaches, has been trenchantly criticised for its conservatism, narrow agenda, stereotyped sets of issues and problems, and its reliance on simplistic arguments and reasoning. Attention has been drawn to crucial, key assumptions underlying much of bioethical discourse, such as the reliance on an individualistic and 'logocentric' perspective, which takes for granted the central role of a thinking, all-powerful subject whose singular task is to formulate and solve through the exercise of reason the main antinomies of modern culture and society.[5]

These criticisms are in fact widely applicable not just to bioethics but to modern ethical thought in general. It is widely assumed in discussions about ethics that to proceed in a systematic fashion it is necessary to identify a problem or dilemma that needs to be solved and then to find solutions to it. It is assumed that ethical problems are solvable and that the solutions can be discovered through the application of rational thought. While these may sound like inoffensive and natural assumptions, in reality they depend on very deep preconceptions about the nature and role of reason and rational argumentation. Furthermore, a major outcome of the logocentrism of ethical thought is that it provides no independent standpoint from which medicine or science can be subject to critique. The object of criticism becomes the standard of criticism. This is one of the reasons for the deep conservatism of much of modern ethical thought.

The central values attributed to individual autonomy—the appeal to the universal abstract principles, the search for definitive 'solutions' to ethical 'dilemmas', the emphasis on outcomes rather than processes—also affirm and support prevailing cultural assumptions. Take the example of medicine again. Dominant approaches to ethics take autonomy, the individual subject, freedom—understood in a historically limited sense of the individual in isolation—as key values. Arguments often presented as 'radical' argue for the legalisation of euthanasia, the killing of disabled persons (including infants and elderly people), the application of genetic techniques to manipulate the genome to increase or improve physical capacity, unrestrained research into stem cells, etc. In many cases these arguments are no more than apologies for the prevailing technological regime. However, of greater importance than this is that they comprehensively set the agenda for all ethical debate. The conclusion that is reached in any particular case makes little difference because the damage has already been done: the task of ethical discourse has been reduced to rubber stamping—or refusing to rubber stamp—the conceptual status quo.[6]

The radicalism of these ethical theories is illusory because they disturb little in the status quo. They do not reflect key issues that arise at the level of the lifeworld—the intimate world of experience we inhabit and share with others in our most intimate interactions. They do not engage the fine texture of day-to-day decision-making; the subtle adjustments we make in the continuous flux of communication, in response to our intuitions about the needs of others; the search for personal meaning and clarity about personal goals and relations with others. They omit the diverse richness and complexity both within and between cultures that distinguish our personal and interpersonal lives.

******

The roots of the concepts of ethics that prevail in contemporary Western societies derive largely from the changes in the understanding of the nature and role of reason that occurred during the intellectual movement around the mid-seventeenth century that became known as the European Enlightenment. The basic conviction guiding this great process of ferment and change was the belief, inspired by science, that progress will occur inexorably towards greater knowledge and social and moral improvement as a result of the application of reason.[7]

The older world views that had dominated prior to this time placed more emphasis on religion and metaphysics than on scientific knowledge. Values spheres dominated that were specific to context, connected to individual lifeworlds, and which linked moral practical elements to private and social life. Practical questions depended on socially integrated contexts of life and were not thought of as purely formal or technical. Similarly, everyday practices in the private and public spheres were not yet formalised and bureaucratised.[8]

The traditional world views had provided unified, shared, stable ways of understanding moral and practical life. In the emerging view of the world, separate regions of discourse and action were distinguished, each of which had its own specific tasks. Science became the major intellectual practice devoted to the search for truth; ethics and jurisprudence assumed the role of carrying out the search for normative rules to guide action; and art became the site for the creation of and reflection on beauty. Each of these areas was the province of 'experts', individuals with specific skills, knowledge and authority whose activities were from now on by and large restricted to a single main field of activity.[9]

One of the major outcomes of the Enlightenment was a differentiation within social life of three relatively autonomous spheres of thought and action: science, morality and art.[10] In the emerging tradition of modernity, the goals of theory were differentiated respectively into the search for truth, the good and the beautiful. The three regions were distinguished as separate, albeit not completely independent. They were linked by their mutual dependence on the overwhelming power of reason.[11]

Perhaps the most crucial innovation of the Enlightenment, however, was the novelty of the concept of reason itself, according to which reason was now seen as a highly refined technical device. Rational thinking was identified with instrumental reason, the kind of thinking that seeks to realise clearly defined outcomes. The application of this reason became the key to all knowledge. From the point of view of the new science, the book of nature, which had now been deciphered, was literally written in mathematical characters.[12] The possibilities and power of reason were considered unlimited. It was to be the tool that would render transparent the obscure complexities of nature and society. The new order was based on some very fundamental assumptions—for example, the 'objectivistic' assumption that the scientist acted as an isolated, monadic, disembodied subject, and that theory merely reflected nature and had freed itself from any contamination with culture.[13] Its notion of reason was 'closed', in the sense that it focused on certain truth, the elimination of ambiguity, the overcoming of uncertainty and the extinction of difference. From now on, one particular kind of reason became the standard for assessing and judging all theoretical claims and empirical phenomena.

Both science and ethics now employed virtually identical notions of the subject. The valuing subject—that is, the subject of ethical discourse—acquired a position and function similar to that of the knowing subject of modern epistemological theory. Both the ethical and the epistemological subjects marked out a centre from which valuations and knowledge—viewed as properties of the subject—could proceed.

Each of the newly defined fields of science, morality and art underwent a process of inexorable systematisation and unification.[14] In the case of morality, the focus became a search for rationally justified rules for good conduct. In fact, morality itself was turned into a process of following universally applicable rules. Approaches to the regulation of conduct that were implicit in the older, now obsolete, world views were progressively rooted out and eliminated as superstition and romanticism, even if they were still employed in foreign cultures, in religious thinking, tribal mythologies and ritualistic practices.

Ethical theories were increasingly justified on the basis of single philosophical methods and general theories of human nature. Morality was given a very narrow focus; it was considered no more than a guide to obligatory action.[15] All dilemmas were assumed to have a rational resolution. All discrepancies in moral views between individuals were to be overcome by the exercise of reason alone. Morality became a matter of formulating rationally based principles of obligatory action. Even where alternatives were proposed—such as attempts to revive the Aristotelian virtues—the newly dominant framework was left intact.[16]

In the new regime, everyday problems—such as my question about whether I should care for my elderly mother—had to be framed within a context that allowed limited options only. If, as a respectable thinker, I wanted to answer this question, I had to adopt one of the conventional possibilities. I had to formulate reasons that addressed such issues as whether she has useful cognitive capacity sufficient to allow her to be regarded as possessing personhood. The cold light of reason demanded that a calculation be undertaken to assess whether her continued life maximised the happiness of the whole society. Religious moralists would try to prove that to care, or not to care, was an obligation that derived from the existence of God. Others would try to identify universal principles that would illuminate or exemplify the specific case of this one woman.

Despite its attraction and apparent successes, the notion of theory as radically independent of culture deeply compromised from the outset the new project of ethics. It undermined its capacity to raise critical questions by making it dependent on instrumental reason. Reflection on the nature of personhood or the role of reason in ethical judgement was largely abolished. The primordial, open, creative process within which subjects and subjectivities crystallise in face-to-face interactions was attenuated, and systematically annulled.[17] The crucial, creative role of the ethical relationship between embodied subjects, pullulating with new meanings, was ignored, and then forgotten.

The Practice of Ethics in Daily Life

The official discourses of ethics do not reflect accurately the everyday experience of ethical practice. In daily life, we make decisions about issues concerning values all the time. Whenever I engage another person, however large or small the interaction, I adjust my conduct in recognition of him or her. Whether I am interacting with a student, a bus driver, a shop keeper or a lover, whether I am engaging in a dinner-time conversation, walking in a crowd or driving on the road, whether I am making decisions about the care of a patient, a child or my elderly mother, I remain acutely attuned to the proximity of others, to the effects on them of my words, my actions, my mere presence. In the continuous flow of these interactions, some mundane and inconsequential, some of great moment and consequence, I carefully adjust my words, my physical actions, my facial expressions, my bodily postures, in recognition of their needs, vulnerabilities and reciprocal responses or lack of response. My daily life is replete with small decisions about my responsibilities for, and effects on, other people.

Some of the decisions I make are explicitly considered and rationally based, and occasionally I may ponder issues of great moment and deep consequence. However, mostly, the ethical content of my life is intuitive and inconspicuous. Ethical discourse in the everyday does not follow rigorous philosophical theories. We do not start from universal, abstract principles or normative rules of conduct and then try to make reality conform to them. We resist and reject strict formulas and dogmatic principles. Instead, we engage in dynamic, open and flexible dialogues with others as we negotiate our way delicately through densely populated fields of often conflicting values. In doing so, we utilise whatever tools are available to us. We appeal to arguments, we engage in discussions, we call up memories, traditions and past conversations, we apply fragments of theory. There are discussions about discussions, and reflections on these discussions. Our conversations may be carried to completion or they may be partial, interrupted and inconclusive. We abide this complex process of bricolage, this strange and mysterious polysemy and ambiguity, without demur or a sense of exception.

Often, to break an impasse we introduce a new element—a joke, a reference to a book we have read or a film we have seen, a past experience. We call on the language to stutter, to enable us to open up a new space of meaning, one that does not forget the weight of the world and the deafness of understandings.[18] We engage in a constant hermeneutics of values and interactions, discovering new landscapes, and problems and truths fitted into one another.[19]

In these practical dialogues that drive our daily lives forward, we do not start from the premise that we are autonomous individuals setting out to establish and then control contact with others. We start from the assumption that we are inexorably and irrevocably enmeshed with others. Our relationships with other people are placed at the very beginning—indeed, even before they become differentiated as relationships. We start from the premise that our very uniqueness lies in our responsibility for others, a responsibility that cannot be passed off to another person, just as I could never have anyone else take my place in death.[20] The uniqueness of my commitment to the other person with whom I am engaged in dialogue establishes my capacity to do only what no-one else can do in my place. This uniqueness and specificity of the 'first person singular' guarantees my freedom.[21] On the other hand, the continuity of my relationships and responsibilities, embedded as they are in thriving, rich and intense dialogues and diverse cultures and ideas, insures against an arbitrary process of relativism or subjectivism.

Neither the starting point nor the process is closed or rigid. The outcomes of the ethical dialogues are often marked by a similar openness and polysemy. In ethics, there are no correct solutions. There is no single point of view or conclusion that distinguishes right conduct from moral error, good from evil. There are no inviolable laws of moral action that command universal obedience: there are only processes with greater or less integrity, with more or less commitment to the openness and creativity inherent in the interpersonal space.

The predominant contemporary philosophical reflections on ethics demand that all thought and meaning are assimilated to a single standard, that they are solid and positive. They assume that reason faithfully reflects a stable, explicable structure of the world. They depend on closed concepts of thinking, subjectivity and dialogue. In our daily ethical practice we implicitly and intuitively dismiss these assumptions and call on very different resources. We work with the richness and fluidity of alterity, of the otherness of other people; we rely on the deep, uncontainable complexity of our responsibility for these others; we engage in open and creative dialogues to establish unique trajectories through the dense congeries of values that compose the plenum of our ethical lives.

Manifesto

The field of ethics is very broad. It covers the full expanse of thought and action directed towards answering the question, 'What should I do?' The agenda of ethics in everyday life is practically inexhaustible. Even the most mundane experience encompasses an ethical component. Our daily lives are textured by small, microethical moments, soaked with ethical resonances: the meeting of eyes in a train, someone giving way in a doorway, a gesture—or lack of a gesture—of kindness in the tea room, mundane interactions with family and friends. The larger-scale experiences of embodiment, puberty, sexuality, childbirth, illness, menopause and old age all have deep ethical content. These experiences may provoke reflections on our personal goals and aspirations, the sources of satisfaction and frustration. From time to time we encounter—and may be perplexed by—dilemmas in respect of which we are called upon to take conscious decisions.

The answers to ethical questions are not limited to universal formulations, principles or formulae. They are complex and heterogeneous, calling on diverse experiences, texts and discourses and often involving dynamic and sometimes unstable compromises. The ethical domain is radically different from that of instrumental or technical rationality. The purpose of instrumental reason is, in any particular case, to define the strategies and techniques that will enable a well-defined goal to be realised. The choice of that goal and the judgement about whether the human and financial costs of achieving it are justified are tasks not for instrumental reason but for ethics, and this can be thought only in ethical terms. In this sense, ethics provides the context for technical thought, and therefore underlies and is presupposed by it.

Ethical thinking differs from the kind of logic commonly assumed in scientific or technical reasoning. Unlike in the latter, for example, the coexistence of opposite and contradictory points of view is acceptable and common in ethics. In scientific thinking we assess a proposition on the basis of its truth value, while in ethics the criterion is not truth but validity. The test of a technical decision or action is its consequences; in ethics, it is the integrity of the process that generated it. A scientific proposition is true if it is cognate with the empirical facts; an ethical process is valid if it arose through a process of open, uncoerced reflection and dialogue. Science aims to narrow and simplify, to specify algorithms to guide action, produce universal principles or rules. Ethics does none of these things: it seeks to enhance respect for and to expand complexity, to acknowledge and value fullness and richness, to create ambiguity and facilitate communication across the boundaries of discourse and cultural life.

The proliferation of ethical moments does not invalidate the elaborate constructions of philosophical ethics; rather, it contextualises them and illuminates their limitations. The large-scale, traditional, global reflections of philosophical ethics help clarify the basic conditions of the possibility of ethical discourse. Furthermore, the codes of behaviour based on conventional rules and principles of action developed for professional and other regional domains of activity are important for ensuring the stability of social relationships. Both the global reflections and the codes of behaviour, however, must be taken together in context and supplemented with the local, micro-ethical domain of experience within which we move and actively make ethical judgements.

When we engage another person in any interchange, we enter into a field of values that is unbounded and indeterminate. We find ourselves not seeking unambiguous solutions to questions concerning the ethical validity of propositions, but negotiating trajectories of values within shared lifeworlds of experience. We proceed incrementally, in infinitesimal steps, as—by trial and error—we explore the contours of this lifeworld. In ethics there is no single, universally valid category of the good; there is not one method. There is an infinity of goods, and many frameworks within which ethical analysis and debate occur.[22] This means that the domain of ethics is much larger and fecund than is generally accepted within the paradigms of conventional ethical theory. It also means that this expanded domain—the microethical domain—is in general not the terrain of spectacular cases involving heroic decisions. Rather, it is the field of day-to-day communication and structured, complex interactions, of subtle gestures and fine nuances of language. In the medical setting it includes the space of the reverberating physician–patient interaction, within which the medical relationship itself acquires a specific form, and deep-seated, often fundamental issues of value are engaged and, at times, thrown into question.[23]

I do not care for my elderly mother who has Alzheimer's disease just because she has useful sentient life or residual personhood, or because she is still capable of happiness, or because killing her does not maximise the happiness or pleasure of the rest of us. I do not care for her because she is of the human species, or because she has a soul, or because we are God's creatures, or because there is a rule or principle or moral law that says that I have to, or because I am or want to be a good person. I care, despite my own failings and hers, because of—or in spite of—my love and resentments, my misgivings and uncertainties, about her and about myself, because of opportunities seized and missed. I care because I have to; because it is the right thing to do; because she is my mother; because caring is a condition of possibility of being human; because I feel compassion and sadness and loss; because I myself am bereft; because I see in the elderly woman the shadows of my own childhood and the poignancy of her past splendour dulled by the ravages of age, and the poignant contemplation of my own future. I care because it is ennobling to care, even in the meanest, most defiled and debased settings, not because victims are inherently noble but because the distinction between carers and the cared for is itself mistaken. I care because there is never a simple dilemma, a single question with an unequivocal answer. I care because I loved this person once and she loved me, because she was the rock on whom I could depend, who provided the starting point from which my own life was launched, because she cared not just for me but also for many others, including my own children. I care because she contains within her the assemblage of meanings and symbols for my life, the trail of a path traced over a long life; because her current predicament cannot be explicated in terms of 'sentience' or 'rationality' or 'quality of life'. I care for her because of her vulnerability and fragility, which is like the vulnerability and fragility she discerned and protected in my children and me. I care for her not because I can string together arguments to make a case. In short, I care with my reason, my emotions, my humanness.

Ethics is a process of dialogue that involves communication across the boundaries of philosophy, personal values, cultural assumptions and political and religious beliefs. Within it, individuals come together to generate and share new meanings, or indeed to define what it is that makes them individuals. Because of these characteristics it is inherently and irrevocably open, fluid and anti-totalitarian.

******

We are all experts in ethics. We live in spaces shaped by ethical considerations. Our face-to-face relationships with others, our deepest and most private emotions, our mundane interactions during the conduct of our daily lives, all involve a multitude of ethical decisions, negotiations and adjustments. In these relationships and private experiences we engage with each other and with the world as embodied subjects, as physical, carnal beings, finite and vulnerable, grappling with our fears and hopes, weaknesses and desires.

One does not have to go to exotic places, seek out extreme circumstances or look for fundamental innovations in science, technology or culture to encounter ethical issues and the challenge of making ethical decisions. In the grey, commonplace continuum of the everyday there is heroism, joy, tragedy, suffering, honour, trust, loyalty, betrayal, altruistic caring and ruthless egoism. There is even evil and good, cynicism and selfless virtue.

In reflecting on our underlying values and aspirations, in taking stock of our lives and planning our futures, in regulating our relationships and locating our places in the plenum of words and things, we draw on the wealth of resources in history and culture, literature, art, religion and philosophy. We engage in mundane or reflective dialogues, we argue and discuss, we respond emotionally and intuitively, and we reason painstakingly. We give weight to the power of reason, which has delivered successes in science, technology, medicine and elsewhere. However, we recognise that reason is not the only, or even the pre-eminent, domain of thought and action in the field of ethics. Rational argument is powerful, but it is not all-powerful.

In the ethical parts of our lives we form the background topography, the multidimensional context, within which we make decisions about how to act, how to intervene in the world, in a strategic manner. Our instrumental actions are focused and single-minded. In ethics, we plot paths through fields of values full of risk and uncertainty. In our technical decisions we look for results and outcomes; in ethics, we accept what is generated by an open, creative process. In ethics, there is no truth and falsity, no unambiguous solutions; there are no right answers. Just because I make a commitment or reach a conclusion does not mean that everyone else has to do the same. On the contrary, plurality and difference, diversity among ethical viewpoints and commitments, only enhance the richness and depth of my own ethical life.

Even in the face of its social function to control behaviour or stabilise social relationships, ethics is, and must be retained as, a domain of radical questioning, of reflection on and scrutiny of deep assumptions and strongly held values. It can be messy, untidy, inconvenient and inconclusive: it should, however, never be allowed to give up its crucial meaning-creating mission.

Notes
1. See Chapter 2.
2. My mother has, in detailed conversations, given permission for me to refer to her condition and the issues it raises.
3. See Chapter 4.
4. I Illich, *Limits to Medicine* (London, Marion Boyars, 1976).
5. See Chapter 1. Also, cf. C Elliott, *A Philosophical Disease: Bioethics, Culture, and Identity* (New York, Routledge, 1999); PA Komesaroff, *Troubled Bodies: Critical Perspectives on Postmodernism, Medical Ethics and the Body* (Melbourne, Melbourne University Press, 1995).

6   See Chapter 2.
7   PA Komesaroff, *Objectivity, Science and Society: Interpreting Nature and Society in the Age of the Crisis of Science* (London, Routledge, 1986; 2008).
8   J Habermas, *The Theory of Communicative Action, Volume 2*, tr. Thomas McCarthy (Boston, Beacon Press, 1981), pp. 324–6.
9   See Chapter 1.
10 J Habermas, *The Philosophical Discourse of Modernity* (Cambridge, MA, MIT Press, 1987), pp. 1–22.
11 J Habermas, *The Theory of Communicative Action, Volume 2*, p. 326.
12 PA Komesaroff, *Objectivity, Science and Society*, pp. 144–8.
13 See PA Komesaroff, *Objectivity, Science and Society*, pp. 11–25; and M Horkheimer and TW Adorno, *Dialectic of Enlightenment* (London, Allen Lane, 1973).
14 See Chapter 1 for a fuller discussion of this subject; cf. also C Taylor, *Sources of the Self* (Cambridge, MA, Harvard University Press, 1989), pp. 76–7.
15 ibid., pp. 89–90.
16 See PA Komesaroff, *Troubled Bodies*, pp. 2–5.
17 See Chapters 1 and 2; M Heidegger, *An Introduction to Metaphysics* (New York, Doubleday, 1959), p. 13. See also Nietzsche, *The Gay Science* (New York, Vintage Books, 1974).
18 E Levinas, 'Revelation in the Jewish Tradition', in EN Dorff and LE Newman, eds, *Contemporary Jewish Theology: A Reader* (Oxford University Press, 1999), pp. 164–78.
19 ibid., p. 170.
20 G Deleuze, *Essays, Critical and Clinical*, tr. DW Smith and MA Greco (Minneapolis, University of Minnesota Press, 1997), pp. 107–114.
21 See A Lingis, *The First Person Singular* (Evanston, North-western University Press, 2007).
22 J-F Lyotard, *Postmodern Condition and Just Gaming* (Minneapolis, University of Minneapolis Press, 1985), pp. 50–9.
23 See Chapter 2.

Part I

Medicine, Postmodernism, Microethics and the Body

CHAPTER 1
Medicine and the Ethical Conditions of Modernity

Two major recent discussions have raised important questions about our understanding of the moral content of the medical sciences: the discussion concerning what used to be called 'practical philosophy' and that focusing on the nature of modernity and its status in the contemporary world. In this chapter I should like to set out some of the themes of these discussions and to consider their implications for medicine.

Discussions about ethics within medicine, like the classical discussions about ethics, depart from the question that anyone seeking to accomplish a practical task must answer: what should I do? Within medical practice, this question is ever-present; furthermore, as is well recognised, depending on the circumstances, it may be subject to a 'technical' as well as an 'ethical' interpretation. All cases, however, involve an appeal to a set of philosophical assumptions and a reliance on a historical tradition. In general, medical practitioners have understood the technical, or scientific, aspect of both their clinical and their research work in conventional, positivistic terms, and in ethical debates they have tended to draw on three classical sources: Kantian moral theory, utilitarianism and Aristotelian ethics. The basis for a questioning of these traditional assumptions arose from a number of theoretical developments, out of which the contemporary debates have emerged.

These developments, which form the background for the discussion here, include the advent of the postempiricist philosophy of science, which scrutinised the process of object formation within scientific theories and emphasised the dependence of the latter on normative considerations and social and cultural variables. They also include the development in sociology, psychology and philosophy of a variety of approaches purporting to offer alternatives to the erstwhile positivistic epistemologies, the most important of which are phenomenology, structuralism and the so-called 'post-structuralist' theories. And they include the enhanced appreciation that has developed of the heterogeneity and complexity of contemporary societies, which in part derives from these theories. Against these tendencies, it should be acknowledged, within the biological sciences themselves there has also occurred in recent years a revival of old mechanistic and reductionist ideas, in the form of sociobiology and the biological reductionism of modern molecular genetics; this is an interesting and important phenomenon in its own right, but will not be considered further here.

Introduction to Microethics

In the last twenty-five years or so, in developed Western societies the ethical content of medicine has come to be understood in terms of the formulations arising from a cluster of theories known as 'bioethics' or 'biomedical ethics'. Although there is some heterogeneity among these theories, they share certain common features—in particular, their commitment to a rational, universalistic ethical theory based on abstract principles. In spite of a superficial plausibility and a wide audience, however, bioethics has proved itself seriously limited, partly because medicine serves a wider variety of ethical goals than can be accommodated in these theories and partly because the assumptions on the basis of which they are constructed are themselves open to question.

Some of the ethical dimensions of medicine are obvious. Medicine can contribute directly to the relief of suffering and pain. By overcoming or mitigating the effects of disease and physical disability that have hitherto been limiting and have compromised the range of available choices, it can help to release us from the limitations imposed by our biological facticity. In individual instances, moreover, conflicts may arise that demand decisions regarding issues involving traditional moral values such as justice or the sanctity of human life. On the other hand, it is well recognised that the practical applications of medicine are limited and distorted by social conditions—by the facts of poverty and wealth, of impotence and power—and that the outcomes of medical knowledge and know-how are not unambiguously beneficent. Indeed, it has been argued trenchantly that the development of modern medicine has been associated with some profoundly malign social consequences[1], including the degradation of intimate and meaning-endowing human experiences into mere technical events[2], and the loss of personal autonomy.[3] In any case, it is clear that ethics is not merely adventitious with respect to medicine, affixed to it after the fact by philosophical experts. Ethics and medicine are intertwined; medicine, as Edmund Pellegrino once put it, is 'a practice of ethics'.

There is another sense in which medicine reveals itself as a practice of ethics. Every clinical relationship consists of a continuous series of ethical events, each of infinitesimal dimension and often inconspicuous to the participants. The doctor within the clinical interaction is constantly faced with the ethical decision about what she should do. How, for example, should she ask this difficult or potentially intrusive question? How should she palpate the abdomen of this man in pain? How should she express the diagnosis of lung cancer to this elderly woman? Of course, there is nothing remarkable about questions of this kind, which are familiar to every clinician. In the flow of the clinical interaction they occur frequently, arising momentarily and being responded to in the ongoing process of communication. They demand ethical decisions, even if those decisions may be made in an intuitive manner. The character of the response may take many forms: it may involve a particular choice of words or manner of delivering those words, or it may be embodied in the pitch of the voice, the length of the pause or the softness of the touch. It will, of course, in turn evoke a response in the patient, to which a further adjustment by the doctor will be made. I admit that this pattern of response and counter-response is a long way from the more familiar processes of ethical argumentation; however, its irreducible ethical content is undeniable and, what is more, it is of crucial importance with respect to the clinical outcomes.

This constant process by which ethical issues arise, are dealt with in the course of the interaction and subsequently pass away, I call the 'microethical structure' of medicine. It is important to recognise the microethical domain because it allows us to describe what doctors and patients actually do, from an ethical perspective. It shifts the focus of ethical discourse about medicine to an analysis of the processes of moral decision-making in the clinical encounter and it makes it possible for us to undertake an anatomy of the ethical interaction in broader terms. It brings into visibility many issues that are inaccessible to the conventional viewpoints of biomedical ethics. Finally—and, of particular importance—it can provide a powerful tool for analysing the complexity of the clinical process and contributing to its further development.

Despite its central importance, the microethical aspect of medicine—and indeed, what might be called the 'sociology of moral action' in medicine—has been very much neglected from the theoretical point of view. The reasons for this are complex: they include the influence of the cultural tradition and the absence of adequate tools to deal with the phenomena that arise. Indeed, despite its straightforward appearance, the concept of microethics involves some very radical claims, which entail a fundamental departure from many of the assumptions on which philosophical ethics has been built. For the perspective of microethics to be accepted, these claims need to be stated and justified in full; and, in addition, the overall utility of the theoretical approach needs to be demonstrated.

Microethics is an important component of both clinical medicine and research. This does not, however, imply that it exhausts the entire ethical content of clinical relationships. It must be understood in the wider context mentioned above—of the social and cultural structures within which the ethical interactions occur and of the philosophical tradition that may be brought to bear in reflecting on ethical and even epistemological issues at a higher level of abstraction. The ethical dimension of medicine is heterogeneous and multifaceted. To understand it we must have access to a theory that can accommodate this diversity and respond to contemporary cultural developments.

Ethics and the Enlightenment

Modern reflections on ethics in medicine from the Western perspective derive in large part from the project in ethics that had its origins in the European Enlightenment around the mid-seventeenth century. The basic conviction that has guided this project has been the belief, inspired by science, that in an unlimited, universal and inexorable way, progress will occur towards greater knowledge and social and moral improvement. Inherent in this vision, furthermore, is the confidence that this progress will be generated and protected by the application of reason.

The Enlightenment provided the nascent project of the Galilean theory of nature with a definitive, systematic elaboration. The goals of science were articulated clearly and succinctly. Science was understood to be a critical part of a social project of universal scope and unlimited application; its telos was nothing less than the liberation of mankind through the complete mastery and domination of both external and internal nature. For almost 200 years, this expansive—and perhaps somewhat immodest—objective provided the goal that guided the aspirations of scientists, philosophers, social theorists and political activists.

Ethical thinking was also brought under this project. The goals of philosophical ethics became very similar to those of science. Ethics and freedom were now coterminous. As for science, the goal of ethical thought was human liberation. It also aimed to abolish doubt and to discover fixed laws that could guarantee certain truth. To realise the goal of human liberation, both the achievements and the methods of science were to be applied universally for the development of society. This objective was as important for moral sceptics like La Mettre as it was for utilitarians like Helvetius, materialists like Diderot or 'idealists' like Kant. For ethics, this meant that a single system of thought had to be sought that was capable of embracing all ethical values, or, at least, of providing a method for the resolution of ethical problems.

As a result, in ethics, as in science and art, there was a powerful tendency to systematisation and unification.[4] In the case of ethics and morality, the task was defined as the search for a rational justification of rules for good conduct. Indeed, morality itself became understood as a process of following rules, usually of universal application. This search for a single principle to guide action became a key feature of modern moral philosophy. Older approaches to ethics and morality that had previously commanded wide acceptance, such as the foundational role of the virtues, or the recognition that there is a number of quasi-autonomous goods, were discounted. In the same way, the role of the philosopher was defined very narrowly. As with the great philosophical theorists of ethics, the philosopher's job was now to identify a procedure or set of procedures that would generate good actions or propositions.

The implications of these assumptions for contemporary ethical theory can be clearly seen in the two major schools of bioethical thought: utilitarian and deontological ethics. Both of these are firmly located in the Enlightenment tradition of philosophical ethics. They share the key assumptions mentioned above; in particular, they share a commitment to the elaboration of universally valid principles through the application of reason and they share an assumption of an objectivistic conception of values. These features constitute the basis both for the ongoing appeal of these theories and, as we shall see, of their main shortcomings.

Critical Responses
The modern tradition of ethics has attracted vehement criticism almost from the beginning. The philosophical interrogations of Hegel, Kierkegaard, Nietzsche, Heidegger and others raised doubts about the ethical project of modernity, although they failed to supplant it. In modern ethics, and in medical ethics in particular, various approaches have come to exist outside the utilitarian and Kantian mainstreams of normative ethics; some of these draw on phenomenology, some on the Marxian tradition, some on a revival of the ideas of Aristotelian ethics. These critical tendencies in fact are profoundly important for our understanding of clinical medicine and research because they both highlight the deficiencies of bioethics and suggest the possibility of alternative theoretical strategies.

A useful way to approach the modern critiques of ethical theory is to consider Hegel's critique of Kant's moral philosophy. This is because the work of the latter contains the most rigorous and complete embodiment of the Enlightenment project and that of the former its most telling interrogation. Hegel made three particularly potent criticisms of Kant: he charged that Kant's morality amounts to little more than an 'empty formalism', that it issues in an 'abstract universalism' and that, as a result, it is condemned to impotence.

Hegel argued that the formalistic approach taken by Kant prevented any concrete content being given to duties and maxims. As a result, he claimed, Kant's conclusions are either tautologous or, worse, they may actually sanction conduct that is clearly unconscionable. In the Kantian context, the moral viewpoint in general admits of normative statements—that is, statements that prescribe rules of conduct at a high level of generality—that arise in rational debate; however, it excludes evaluative statements about the good life and the chance of realising it in the existing culture. Hegel argues that 'the real bond of moral duty depends on the way in which duties bear on people's social roles and relationships in the ethical life of a rational social order'.[5] In other words, moral philosophy remains limited to a formal theoretical standpoint and cannot make contact with the deeper, underlying substrata of social interactions that constitute the deeper reality of what Hegel refers to as 'ethical life'.[6]

Related to this, Hegel argues that Kantian ethics is dependent on a commitment to an 'abstract universalism'. As a matter of general principle, it ignores the particular context, including the social and emotional contexts, in which problems arise. The concept of duty becomes not just the 'empty thought of universality' but moves to exclude or dominate all other relations.[7] As a consequence of these commitments to empty formalism and abstract universalism, Hegel concludes, morality is impotent with respect to the accomplishment of the good. Because moral acts are restricted to those which are in accordance with 'the law', the good is left 'only in the idea, in representation'. Morality dichotomises reason and experience: it is incapable of making the transition from the pure 'ought' to the 'is'.[8]

These three criticisms by Hegel against Kant are telling ones for contemporary bioethical thought. In all its major variants, bioethics is committed to the distinction between the normative and the evaluative. The whole purpose of ethics, as conceived by the bioethical thinkers, is to provide a machinery for analysing and resolving conflicts and dilemmas through the application of rational modes of thought. Rational argument is the exclusive medium within which conflict resolution takes place. In one sense this approach is unobjectionable: rational discourse is, for example, clearly preferable to violence. However, its main problem is its omission—previously referred to—of the level of ethical life. For Hegel, ethical life—which he calls *Sittlichkeit*—is an essential part of the social world. It is the stratum of social life that is organised into institutions and experienced by individuals in their daily interactions. It is the 'living shape of organic totality' of a community.[9] It thus has a double aspect: it is both a differentiated and structured social order and a subjective disposition within that order; or, put differently, it is both a 'relation between many individuals' and the 'form of the concrete subject'.[10]

Bioethics is also vulnerable in relation to the second criticism—that of abstract universalism. The emphasis on normative ethics limits the ability of bioethical theories to consider not just the contexts within which norms are applied but the intersubjective processes through which moral actions are effected in general. What is omitted here is not merely analyses of individual cases, but also the performative aspects of moral interchanges—that is, the manner in which they are actually realised in practice, according to which the ethical meanings of individual communicative acts are located and oriented. Finally, there is also a strong case that bioethics is in practical terms impotent—that is, that it is incapable of effecting the transition from theory to action. This is a more controversial point; here, we shall say no more than that despite all the debate it has generated about public policies, there appears to be no evidence that biomedical ethics has beneficially affected medical practice at the level of the clinic.[11]

Hegel's identification of key problems within Kant's practical philosophy facilitated the development of a variety of alternative approaches to moral theory. In the contemporary context, two of the most important of these are the so-called neo-Aristotelian theories and the discourse ethics of Jürgen Habermas, to which we merely advert briefly here.

Habermas seeks to continue the tradition of Kantian ethics, albeit with modifications to overcome the difficulties revealed by Hegel. Like Kant, he is committed to the possibility of universal moral principles, and he continues the search for a method for establishing normative rules through rational argumentation. He departs from the latter—and, for that matter, from the rest of the philosophical tradition—however, by shifting the emphasis decisively towards 'communicative action'—that is, social action directed towards communicative, rather than primarily technical or strategic, ends. For Habermas, communicative action, and specifically linguistically mediated interactions, constitutes the basic motor of the social processes. In accordance with this basic perspective, his ethical theory is intended precisely to reformulate the Kantian project in intersubjective terms, as an analysis of moral argumentation. This approach leads to some very strong conclusions, such as his statement of a 'universal principle' of moral action, which, he claims, has binding force with respect to communicative interactions in general. In addition, it succeeds in shifting the focus of the traditional moral discourse to the moral 'lifeworld', to use a terms of Husserl's employed frequently by Habermas—that is, to the interactive context within which moral decisions are made; a context that, in the medical context, ought to include the microethical domain.

Unfortunately, however, the moral lifeworld for Habermas is curiously partial and attenuated. His commitment to the search for universal normative principles and his decision to restrict moral phenomena to conflicts in linguistically mediated discursive contexts prevents his theory from gaining access to the interactive contexts within which the great bulk of our ethical experiences occur. Indeed, it is precisely one of Habermas' defining criteria of moral phenomena that they are disengaged from, and therefore cannot be contaminated by, the local conventions of particular forms of life. Accordingly, his theory ultimately prescinds from the real (linguistic and nonlinguistic) context of interaction. This condemns it to a very limited field of application—and certainly excludes it from making a contribution at the level of the clinical interchange. As a result, Habermas' discursive reconstruction of Kantian ethics itself ultimately results in a disappointing impotence.

A quite different approach is taken by the so-called 'neo-Aristotelian' philosophers. Like Habermas, they set out to provide an ethics appropriate to the modern age that circumvents the abstractions and formalism in the extant tradition that Hegel exposed so powerfully. However, whereas Habermas attempts to develop a procedural approach to morality by radically separating the right and the good, they seek to resurrect a universalistic ethics of the good that appeals to supreme goods transcending all particular forms of life. For them, although ethical judgements are understood to be dependent on specific contexts and circumstances, they are nonetheless not guided by the classical moral question 'What ought I to do?', but by the more encompassing question 'What is the good life?' Thus, Charles Taylor seeks to identify 'constitutive goods', which are underlying moral sources on the basis of which not only individual goods but the motivation to do and be good arises[12]; similarly, Alasdair MacIntyre, in a classical Aristotelian fashion, outlines a range of 'virtues', the possession of which enables us to achieve specific goods.[13]

This perspective, like that of discourse ethics, offers a trenchant critique of the dominant traditions of moral thought. Further, it emphasises the need for an exploration of 'the order in which we are set as a locus of moral sources', an order 'that is only accessible through personal, hence "subjective" resonance'.[14] On the other hand, as Habermas has argued, it is subject to major problems, which include its alleged commitment to ahistoricism and methodological individualism[15], and its inability to deal with the pluralism of modern societies.

From the point of view of medicine, neo-Aristotelianism undoubtedly has much to offer. However, in view of the variety of the cultural perspectives of individual doctors and patients, and the multiplicity of purposes that medicine can serve, serious questions are raised about the claim that competing ways of life can be arranged hierarchically. Furthermore, at the local or microethical level, it is rare that values guiding decision-making can be directly linked to constitutive goods, and attempts to do so tend to be not only theoretically implausible but also often practically restrictive.

The Postmodernist Challenge to the Project of Modernity

While the 'Enlightenment project of ethics' was being subjected to a barrage of criticisms and alternatives, important cultural changes were occurring in the society as a whole—changes with the capacity to produce a profound, direct effect on both the theory of morality and the practice of medicine. The integrity of the project of modernity itself was being thrown into question and its most fundamental assumptions subjected to a searing critique. For some, these changes amount to an epochal transition: from modernity to postmodernity. Now it is important to note that the nature of 'postmodernism' and its status as a concept remain controversial.[16] Nonetheless, there are certain novel features of the contemporary cultural configurations of developed Western societies that demand to be acknowledged. These include a rejection of the commitment to certain knowledge and the search for an irrefutable foundation for truth. They include a particular emphasis on the need for an ongoing reflection on, and awareness of, the process of the generation of cultural products, including, in particular, of knowledge itself. And they include a rejection of the 'grand narrative' as historically obsolete—especially the great cultural constructions of 'humanity', of 'the proletariat', of 'womankind', of 'beauty', of 'truth' and of the project of universal 'liberation'.[17] The central subject from which truth and knowledge have flowed for 300 years is abolished; and the notion of a single totalising reason as the organon, guarantor and guardian of knowledge is abandoned.[18]

From the point of view of postmodernity, in the place of knowledge (in the singular) are now discourses (in the plural)[19], which can proliferate and may be incommensurable, but nonetheless are not excluded from the demands of rigour and complexity. In the place of reason there are only 'reasons'.[20] In the place of the central, potent subject is the 'decentred' subject, no longer structurally disengaged from the social processes that constituted it, but implicated within them and constantly being generated by them. The postmodern world, then, is a place of infinite variety and diversity. In it there are no fixed, unchallengeable criteria for judgement. Instead, contending perspectives are fostered and encouraged. This world is a place of radical freedom, in which the existential choices extend not just to the external circumstances of one's life but to the nature of one's subjectivity itself. The postmodern person is thus contingent; this is, so it is claimed, the shared experience of the contemporary world.[21]

While postmodern theory has been applied to art and art criticism and to other aspects of culture in the computer age, it must be observed that it has been applied to a much more limited extent to ethical theory, and almost not at all to medical ethics in respect of either clinical practice or research. Nonetheless, the overall arguments are as compelling here as they are with respect to aesthetics. The dissolution of aesthetic norms has meant a transformation in the nature of artistic creation. No longer is art subject to the category of beauty—which, as the principle guiding the production of artistic works, itself only came into existence with the Renaissance.[22] Instead, art can now subserve a wide variety of aesthetic interests, 'an infinity of purposes', as Husserl said in another context. It can now challenge many of the distinctions formerly assumed to be inviolable—the distinction between art and everyday life, and between the high and the popular cultures, for example—and it can discover new tasks and experiment with new methods of creation. Similarly, in postmodern society, ethics is concerned with a wide range of issues regarding values, the nature of the good life and how one should behave in relation to other people both in general and in specific circumstances. Here, too, there has been a growing recognition that society is a battleground for contending value systems. As Max Weber—one of the great theorists of modernity—put it: 'forty years ago there existed a view that of the various possible points of view one was correct. Today, this is no longer the case; there is a patchwork of cultural values'.[23]

Just as in the field of aesthetics there is no single category of beauty that can provide a universally applicable aesthetic norm, so also in ethics there is no longer a single, universally valid category of the good. There is not one good but an infinity of goods; there is not one method but a multiplicity of discursive frameworks, within which ethical analysis and debate can occur.[24] Once again, great systems are opposed rather than sought, and diversity is promoted and celebrated. The task of ethics is no longer to define the nature of the good, or duty, or 'the ends of man', and much less to derive irrefragable principles for correct action. Rather, it is to uncover the nature of ethical values and the process of value creation; it is to examine existing concepts and to expose their hidden assumptions; and it is to challenge the hegemony of existing value systems and so to expand the possibilities for ethical action.

An Anatomy of the Ethical Interchange in the Clinic

From this brief survey of the deficiencies of the contemporary bioethical constructions and the cultural changes that have characterised late modernity, some proposals regarding the understanding of medicine and its ethical content can be put forward. These proposals must recognise several important facts. First, given the diversification and differentiation of the project of ethics in the 'postmodern' world, it must be accepted that the field of ethical phenomena can be limited neither by the search for universal norms nor by the pursuit of the good life. Rather, evaluative activities that are not specifically orientated towards the good have become equally valid components of the ethical domain. Secondly, not all interactive behaviour with ethical content occurs in the context of theoretical discourse aimed at generating universally valid norms. While moral action may always carry some normative content, this may be only 'local', in the sense of being restricted to the immediate context of interaction rather than extending to the social group or the society as a whole. Thirdly, the importance of this local aspect of ethical interactions—that is, the microethical aspect—needs to be recognised and its nature examined. It is apparent that, in addition to providing the actual site at which moral interactions occur and at which new practical interventions are introduced and tested, the microethical domain has a substantive content and structure of its own. And fourthly, the relationship between the microethical structures and the larger-scale structures of ethical organisation in the society need to be elaborated and their dynamics described; in other words, we need to study the interchanges between the ethical structures of the lifeworld (to use Husserl's term again) and those of the social and cultural system as a whole. In particular, medicine must be understood as a complex set of value-laden practices embedded in the social and cultural structures of an evolving society.

Medical practice, and its ethical dimensions in particular, are therefore complex and heterogeneous, but they nonetheless have a definite structure. There are at least three strata which I call the 'global', the 'regional' and the 'local'. Viewed from the broadest perspective, there are *global* structures that are common to every interaction with ethical content. These have the status of conditions of possibility of ethical discourse; they include procedural principles of universal application, such as Habermas' discursive reformulation of the categorical imperative (with the understanding that the ethical field be expanded to include non-linguistically mediated phenomena). I have said that these principles are 'universal', on the basis of their putative transcendental status, although this should be qualified with the possibility that they may be culturally specific and therefore subject to variation between societies with widely different cultures and traditions. In a functional sense, these principles may be regarded as constitutive of the ethical interaction per se and are not different for medicine than for any other interactive context.

At the next level, there are the ethical forms that derive from the social groups to which the participating individuals belong. In terms of the interaction, these can be characterised in relation to the specific discursive forms that are deployed in the exchange. In any particular case, there may be several discourses acting simultaneously. Furthermore, the possibility exists of at least some of these having the capacity to reflect on the others—to act, that is, as a 'metadiscourse'; this is precisely the case with the medical discourse. Imperatives can be derived at this level, but they are *regional* rather than universal; their applicability is restricted to the discursive frameworks in which they are embedded. Functionally, these regional imperatives, therefore, are of a regulative kind. In the medical context, the regional level refers to the particular discourses that are employed in clinical interactions—the 'biological', the 'social', the 'psychological', the 'therapeutic' and so on—and to the specific requirements that emerge from the structures of the particular relationships that are established. Here it is important to recognise that each discourse may be associated with a set of moral imperatives of its own, and that these may not all be consistent; at this level, therefore, there is a proliferation of moral values, each with a purely regional sphere of applicability.

Finally, at the *local* level, there are the interactive practices that occur within the constraints of the lifeworld. This is the level of microethics—in functional terms, the substantive level of the ethical relationship. Here, the interchange proceeds incrementally, with constant reference and responsiveness to its specific circumstances and the changing local context. It is subject to the contingencies of individual interchanges, and because there are many degrees of freedom, the processes may be highly unpredictable. The constitutive principles and the regulative imperatives of the global and the regional structures continue to operate here; however, at this level, there are no endogenous rules to guide conduct along a predetermined path and there are no ultimate criteria by which actions can be retrospectively judged. Any 'ethic' here can be no more than a local procedural one—for example, along the lines of an 'ethic of responsibility'—but it must be remembered that even this will be devoid of teleological content.

The microethical domain, despite its unavoidable presence in any ethical interaction, has been remarkably neglected in theoretical discussions about ethics. Because of this lack of study, at this stage a limited amount can be said about its structures. Nonetheless, it is apparent that the microethical domain does have structures of its own; these are substantially the structures of interpersonal interaction in the lifeworld. Some of the characteristic features of the microethical domain have already been described. Its phenomena are continuous, in the sense of constituting an infinite array of infinitesimal events. Each of these is contingent on the current state of the interactive context—because the latter is itself subject to a great many degrees of freedom, this makes microethical phenomena inherently unpredictable and subject to extreme variations with respect to initial conditions. Within the microethical domain, each subject may speak with different voices at different times; this adds further to its heterogeneity and complexity.

The three domains that constitute the ethical structure of medicine are of course interdependent. The global domain is logically prior, in the sense of constituting conditions of possibility for any ethical relationship. On the other hand, the microethical domain is factually and practically prior, since all ethical behaviour passes through this realm, and is therefore subject to its structural constraints, including its uncertainties: it is the interface between interpersonal interactions and the remainder of the ethical apparatus; it functions as the domain within which values arise and are tested, and ethical pathologies manifest themselves.

******

In the light of contemporary debates about the nature of ethics and society, some assumptions about morality and morally motivated actions must be reassessed. In particular, we must seriously consider the possibility of an ethical theory that is not only structurally committed to heterogeneity and diversity, but is also radically disengaged from any unitary notion of the good.

Although for some, this conclusion may appear somewhat disquieting, it would seem unavoidable if the achievements of modernity are to be taken seriously and the rich, multifaceted nature of the medicine to which it has given rise is to be recognised. In addition, as we shall see, it provides a much-needed tool for analysing in detail the moral content of both clinical medicine and medical research, for exposing underlying cultural assumptions and thereby for deepening our appreciation of the nature of medicine.

Notes

1. I Illich, *Limits to Medicine* (London, Marion Boyars, 1976).
2. ibid., p. 26.
3. J Ehrenreich, ed., *The Cultural Crisis of Modern Medicine* (London, Monthly Review Press, 1978).
4. C Taylor, *Sources of the Self* (Cambridge, MA, Harvard University Press, 1989), pp. 76–7.
5. AM Wood, *Hegel's Ethical Thought* (Cambridge, Cambridge University Press, 1990), p. 132.
6. GWF Hegel, *Philosophy of Right* (Oxford, Oxford University Press, 1952), pp. 89–90.
7. GWF Hegel, *Early Theological Writings*, tr. TM Knox (Philadelphia, University of Pennsylvania Press, 1971), p. 212.
8. ibid.
9. GWF Hegel, *Natural Law*, tr. TM Knox (Philadelphia, University of Pennsylvania Press, 1975), p. 108.
10. AM Wood, *Hegel's Ethical Thought*, p. 196.
11. See Chapter 2.
12. C Taylor, *Sources of the Self*; see Chapter 3.
13. A MacIntyre, *After Virtue* (London, Duckworth, 1987), ch. 14.
14. C Taylor, *Sources of the Self*, p. 510.
15. J Habermas, *Justification and Application* (Cambridge, MA, MIT Press, 1993), ch. 3.
16. J-F Lyotard, *The Postmodern Condition: A Report on Knowledge* (Manchester, Manchester University Press, 1986); J Baudrillard, *Simulations* (New York, Semiotext(e), 1983); A Heller and F Feher, *The Postmodern Political Condition* (London, Polity, 1988); F Jameson, 'Postmodernism, or the Cultural Logic of Late Capitalism', *New Left Review*, 146, 1984: 53–93.
17. J-F Lyotard, *The Postmodern Condition*, pp. 31ff.
18. J-F Lyotard, *The Postmodern Condition*; J Derrida, 'The Ends of Man', in *Margins of Philosophy* (London, Harvester Press, 1982).
19. P Murphy, 'Postmodern Perspectives and Justice', *Thesis 11*, 30, 1991: 118.
20. J-F Lyotard, 'An Interview with Jean-Francois Lyotard', W van Reijen and D Veerman, *Theory, Culture and Society*, 5, 1988: 278.

21 A Heller, 'The Contingent Person and the Existential Choice', The Philosophical Forum XXI, 1989–90 (1–2).
22 A Heller, *Renaissance Man* (New York, Schocken Books, 1981), pp. 252–3.
23 M Weber, 'The Meaning of "Ethical Neutrality" in Sociology and Economics', in *The Methodology of the Social Sciences* (New York, The Free Press, 1949), pp. 3–4.
24 J-F Lyotard, *Postmodern Condition and Just Gaming* (Minneapolis, University of Minneapolis Press, 1985), pp. 50–9.

Chapter 2

From Bioethics to Microethics
The Need to Return Ethical Debate to the Clinic

It is midnight in the emergency room of a country hospital. A patient is carried in by four attendants. He is angry and aggressive, shouting obscenities and struggling vigorously. It transpires that he is a prisoner in a local jail and that the attendants are warders. One of them claims that he has been behaving irrationally and needs medical attention. When approached, however, the patient becomes even more hostile and refuses to cooperate in any way.

From the point of view of the bioethicist, the issues here seem clear. They include the degree of autonomy the patient can exercise in these circumstances—which will depend on the fact of whether or not he is 'competent'—balanced against the doctor's obligations of non-maleficence and beneficence; questions of justice, including the fairness and even-handedness of the treatment of this particular individual, may also be relevant. From the point of view of the clinician, however, the problem appears very different. Putting aside issues about the likely specificity of this perspective for particular cultural groups within contemporary, developed Western societies, the key ethical question is not 'How autonomous is this patient?' but 'How are we going to communicate with him?' At the level of the clinic, the task is to determine how to approach this person, for whom doctors and hospitals are likely to be regarded with some suspicion, in order to establish a relationship that will allow the clinical process to proceed; this includes, of course, a decision regarding any immediate medical assessment that is necessary and how this might be performed. The task, in other words, is first of all to talk to the patient, to gain his trust: to engage him in the particular context of the clinic.

******

The emergency room again, late at night. The patient is a middle-aged, non-English-speaking man, surrounded by his large, very concerned family. He complains, loudly and repeatedly, of abdominal pain. However, he refuses to allow anyone to touch his abdomen in order to perform the appropriate physical examination, which he clearly regards as unnecessary.

Once again, the perspectives of the bioethicist and the clinician diverge. For the former, as previously, the case presents a relatively straightforward ethical problem. Is the patient legitimately exercising his autonomy in refusing to let you examine him? If he is, there is in all probability little else to be said. For the latter, however, while the problem is indeed an ethical one, it is of a somewhat different kind. Here, the issue concerns the form and texture of the communication between the doctor and the patient, having regard both to the cultural and to the personality factors at work. From the clinical viewpoint, the question is formulated not in terms of 'autonomy' but practically, in terms of the most appropriate way to approach the patient, to talk with him, to allay his fears and to establish the common ground on which mutual decisions can be taken.

This chapter seeks to examine the difference between the approach to the ethical problems in medicine developed by contemporary bioethics and that inherent in the practice of clinical medicine.

Medical Ethics Today

There has been in recent years an explosion of interest in medical ethics. The dilemmas of modern medicine are now widely and vigorously discussed in the popular media, in the community at large and in the medical literature. The curricula of almost all medical schools incorporate at least some teaching on the subject of the ethical issues associated with medical practice, and biomedical ethics has become a respectable field of study in its own right. There are at least ten international journals devoted exclusively or predominantly to the field; there are graduate courses and dedicated research institutes devoted to defining and pursuing its problems. It is perhaps not too much of an exaggeration to say that bioethics now constitutes a substantial academic industry.

The enhanced interest in medical ethics represents a response to a perception in the community that medicine has somehow lost touch with its original purposes—that it has been transformed into an efficient instrument for achieving technical goals, with little regard to their human or social implications.[1] The development of rigorous methods of reflection on current practices, furthermore, has indeed gone some of the way to meeting that concern and, undeniably, has thereby produced some beneficial consequences. For example, at least partially as a result of these debates, doctors have become more aware of the conceptual issues implicit in decisions that they previously often made without deep consideration, and they have developed skills in critical reflection and argumentation. The medical profession in general has become more sensitive to community attitudes. At the same time, in the community generally, the complexity of medical practice has become more widely appreciated.

However, reflection on the ethical problems of medicine and biology has come to be largely dominated by a series of assumptions, conventions and imperatives regarding the formulation of the questions to be considered and the methods of argument. This has given rise to some disquiet among many practising clinicians, because the body of thought in question—to which we shall refer in general as 'bioethics'—often appears to present the ethical discussions as abstract and divorced from the real concerns of doctors and patients, with many of the most important issues being obscured or passed over. Consequently, the ethical analysis does not always contribute to the actual decision-making process. Furthermore, and possibly more importantly, both practising clinicians and their patients often feel at a disadvantage—that they are in some way out of their depth—when talking about ethical issues, which are thus left to be dealt with in the technical domain of the philosophers.

There is a growing, if still incipient, recognition of the deficiencies of bioethics among both the medical and the philosophical communities. Indeed, there is now a substantial body of writing reflecting critically on bioethics and its philosophical foundations. This literature includes specific analyses from within bioethics itself[2], critiques by practising clinicians[3] or by philosophers working in the field of the ethics of medical practice but outside the paradigms of bioethics proper[4], and reflections of a more global nature on the foundations of ethical theory.[5] Among the many criticisms that are advanced in these discussions are the claims that bioethics reflects and reinforces the values of a particular cultural perspective within Western societies, that it lacks a reliable theoretical foundation, and that many of its arguments are circular. The question is also raised of the proper relationship between bioethics, which is concerned with complex issues covering many disciplines, and philosophical ethics, in its various forms, which has often been assumed—without sufficient justification, it is claimed—to provide a theoretical framework for the entire discourse.

It is not a concern of this chapter to provide a detailed critique of bioethics, or even to offer an exhaustive list of the many standpoints from which it has been subjected to scrutiny. Instead, in what follows, some of its fundamental deficiencies will be outlined and some suggestions will be made regarding possible future directions for ethical reflections on medical practice. My claim is that bioethics is deficient because it is unable to provide an adequate account of day-to-day decision-making in medicine, as a result of which it cannot provide any substantial guidance for medical practice. I argue that this is not an accidental circumstance and cannot be blamed merely on the development of a 'biomedical establishment' made up of philosophers, lawyers, theologians and sociologists rather than of practising clinicians.[6] Rather, the problem has its roots in the historical tradition from which contemporary philosophical ethics arose. It manifests itself not just in the conclusions of specific arguments but also, more fundamentally, in the ways in which the objects of the discipline are formulated and in the strategies of argumentation that are employed.

The subjects covered by the bioethical literature are already familiar and are of substantial public interest. This apparent familiarity is itself largely a product of the bioethical culture and indicates one of its most pernicious effects, which has been to circumscribe the domain of objects that can legitimately be considered under the rubric of 'ethical debate'. Terms like 'euthanasia', 'confidentiality', 'autonomy' and 'paternalism', 'genetic engineering' and 'in-vitro fertilisation' are not only well known today and easily employed in ordinary language, but have come to be identified as the whole subject matter of medical ethics. At least in the field of medicine, an array of categories—which are exhaustively analysed in the literature—has replaced the more humble but less easily classifiable process of grappling with ethical questions as they arise in the daily course of social life.[7] This testifies to the great power of the language and structure of bioethics—what we might call the 'bioethical discourse'—and the degree to which the assumption of the agenda of bioethics has in fact penetrated everyday life.

The limiting effects of the bioethical discourse in fact go further than this. They determine not just what is considered the appropriate domain of ethical argument, but also the general strategy of argument itself. A question to be analysed from the point of view of its ethical content is usually posed as a dilemma—that is, as a problem in a well-demarcated theoretical field that itself specifies the possible form of the solution. Thus, most commonly, it is postulated that particular choices need to be made from a narrow range of formal possibilities, each of which is associated with both attractive and unattractive implications. The discourse itself is subsequently directed towards guiding our choices and thereby supposedly resolving the dilemma. The effect of this procedure is that the focus is not on the actual process of clinical judgement but on formalised and abstracted representations of medical practice. Its validity and, indeed, that of the criteria of judgement that are incorporated within it, are not themselves subject to critical scrutiny from within the discipline of bioethics; nor could they be, for they are, after all, the conditions of existence of the discourse itself.

For medical ethics, then, not only have the objects of study been circumscribed by the contemporary bioethical discourse, but the methods employed to study them have been limited too. As a result, in respect of at least one aspect of its putative agenda, bioethics has already failed. Instead of opening up practical medicine to the critical instruments of the philosophical tradition, it has imposed a new, limited regime of its own. Instead of achieving an integration between the clinical disciplines and the cultural ones, it has widened the gulf. In the sense that will be explicated below, the practices of working doctors and the philosophical reflection on medicine are further apart than ever.

The underlying problem can be simply stated. The conventional approaches of medical ethics deviate fundamentally from the experiences of everyday medical practice. They are based on a mistaken notion of what medicine is about, a misunderstanding of both the ways in which ethical problems arise at the level of the clinic and the manner in which decisions are taken. The theoretical understanding of medicine, in other words, has to an important extent lost contact with the world of experience it was intended to represent. This is why the discipline itself has a very limited amount to offer practising doctors or their patients.

The major concerns expressed in the public debates about medical ethics ignore many of the most important issues. They ignore, for example, the finely textured and subtle nature of the interaction between doctor and patient and the social context in which it occurs. They ignore the manner in which problems are formulated within this relationship and the ways in which the various possible courses of action are identified. Most importantly, they ignore the delicate ongoing process of negotiation and compromise that characterises human relationships in general and in particular underlies any therapeutic interaction. Put differently, conventional medical ethics is unable to provide an understanding of, and hence a basis for intervention in, the medical lifeworld.

It may be appropriate to emphasise once more at this point that what is being considered here is the mainstream of contemporary bioethics, which comprises a vast body of literature with many contending themes and differences in emphasis. It is not suggested that no analyses have been undertaken of the internal structure of the medical interaction; on the contrary, outstanding contributions have been made to our understanding of this relationship, as has been mentioned above and will be discussed further below.[8]

Moreover, there is no intention to imply that the kinds of dilemmas considered in discussions about medical ethics do not occasionally arise or that the arguments that are employed there are completely irrelevant; indeed, the results of the arguments in the bioethical literature can be both interesting and valuable. However, from the point of view of their potential contribution towards the facilitation or enhancement of actual clinical practice, it must be recognised that such reflections are at best only partial. The vast majority of medical decisions are taken in an ethical environment in the absence of any obvious dilemma. They are made within an organic, ongoing relationship, in the spirit of open dialogue between doctor and patient. Accordingly, medical ethics needs to focus on the practical decision-making context. It must certainly be multidisciplinary—'sociological', 'philosophical', 'psychological' and 'biological'. More importantly, it needs to return to the real roots of medicine itself and to immerse itself in its own proper theoretical objects.

Restoration of the Microethical Domain

Ethical questions in everyday clinical medicine are both more pervasive and more limited than the conventional perspective provided by bioethics would suggest. Crucial ethical issues are involved not just in the great questions of life and death but also in those clinical decisions that at first sight appear to be the simplest and most straightforward. It should be clear here that I am employing a very broad, although historically well founded, notion of the nature of ethics. This notion is encompassed within the classical Kantian formulation of the task of ethics and is especially appropriate for medicine. From the very first contact between doctor and patient to the last interaction that occurs between them, the ethical question about what ought to be done is perpetually and critically at issue. This process includes every aspect of the communicative interaction. It includes the establishment of the implicit goals of the encounter and the taking of the history. It includes the conduct of the physical examination—in itself an extraordinary admixture of ethical and epistemological contents. It includes the choices made in deciding what investigations are to be undertaken and in formulating therapeutic strategies. Ethical decisions are implicated when the meanings of the outcomes are assessed and the community's possible interests in them are considered.

In other words, medical ethics is not just about the dramatic questions that are discussed widely in the popular media or in the philosophical texts. Ethics is what happens in every interaction between every doctor and every patient.

The doctor is involved in a constant stream of choices of an ethical kind, which are made at the local level of his or her interaction with the patient and which bear on its most minute aspects. The accumulation of these microethical decisions, together with the technical decisions with which they are intimately linked, contributes importantly to the final outcome of any particular medical encounter. Arguably—allowing for the context in which the original approach to the doctor is made—medical outcomes depend more on the microethical decisions than on any other factors, including the decisions that may, in relevant circumstances, eventually emerge regarding the more familiar life and death issues. Yet the microethical environment of medicine is rarely discussed in medical courses from the point of view of its constitutive ethical nature[9]; it is virtually never considered in the international bioethics literature or popular debates.

In the clinical interaction, both doctor and patient are engaged in an unbroken continuum of ethical decision-making. In the terms of the physician, there is the manner in which questions are asked of the patient and the responses made to the latter's answers or statements. This includes not only the choice of words but also the manner of their delivery—the tone of the voice, facial expressions and so on. In addition, there is the degree of interest and compassion demonstrated when the more intimate matters are discussed.[10] During the physical examination, there is the general bearing that the doctor adopts and, in particular, the way in which those parts of it in which the patient might feel most vulnerable are conducted. Here, small matters may be very important: the time taken, the communication of commitment and concern, the sensitivity of the touch.

The microethical context also embraces the kind of information given to the patient and the manner in which it is expressed. It includes the way in which the patient's participation in the decision-making process is obtained and the physician's openness to the contributions or suggestions that he or she might make. It includes the formulation of the problem and the decisions that are taken—regarding further investigation, therapy or other strategies—to deal with it. And this is only the beginning. Every aspect of the relationship between doctor and patient is suffused with ethical considerations. Clinical medicine is immanently ethical; within it, the process of ethical judgement is continuous.

As far as the patient is concerned, a very similar situation exists. Here, too, there is a continuous series of ethical decisions that need to be taken. These depend on the relationship that is established with the doctor and they bear mainly on the conditions of the interaction itself. They determine, for example, the degree of openness to the doctor that is adopted, the kind of information that is offered and the detail that is included; they determine the receptiveness to suggestions that might be made regarding underlying causes or lifestyle factors that might be considered contributory; and they determine the readiness to participate in any proposed therapeutic process.

To make this more concrete, consider the example of a young woman attending a clinic complaining of common, non-specific symptoms, including tiredness and malaise, that had been present for a few weeks. Here, to be sure, the usual 'history', 'physical examination' and 'investigations' need to be pursued—with appropriate sensitivity to the culture or ethnicity of the young woman—with the aim of leading to a diagnosis and development of a therapeutic strategy. However, as a moment's reflection will confirm, despite the commonplace, everyday nature of this 'case', even a conversation that is apparently most straightforward raises many delicate and subtle issues. These issues concern the way in which questions are asked and information is sought. For example, how does one gain the trust of a person one has never met before, to such an extent that she will grant access to her most private experiences? How do I ask about the effects of her illness? How should I broach the subject of any specific fears or anxieties she may have had? How do I ask about her sexual experiences, and about contact with drugs or other infective sources? And what about the physical examination? How do I apply the uncompromising, analytical touch of the scientist to someone who is in pain and is undoubtedly frightened and anxious? How do I—under any circumstances—'palpate' a breast, knowing that for the woman her breast is never merely a biological organ stripped of meaning and value. How can I 'perform' a gynaecological examination, which may be painful or frightening or, for some women, be associated with unpleasant or distressing connotations or personal invasion and sexual penetration?

These are all ethical questions that can be answered only when supplemented with the details of the practical discourse that is constituted by the actual interaction. They concern the ways in which we conduct ourselves at the actual point where clinical medicine is realised. They are, indeed, the real material of medical practice.[11]

The microethical issues may seem less spectacular and dramatic than the more familiar bioethical concerns about the possible cessation of life-supporting treatments or the number of cells at which human life begins. Furthermore, from the point of view of many professional ethicists, they lack philosophical interest or even 'ethical significance'; and they are difficult to formulate in terms of established, well-defined ethical categories or dilemmas demanding particular kinds of decisions. However, the microethical considerations and their associated interactions are precisely what constitute the vast bulk of medical practice. More than any other factors, they determine the outcomes of actual clinical encounters. Indeed, clinical practice can only be properly understood and the problems that arise in medical decision-making can only be adequately elucidated once the central and constitutive role of the microethical structure of medicine is recognised. Accordingly, its putative philosophical interest aside, in terms of relevance to the lives of ordinary people, microethics is of pre-eminent importance.[12]

Microethics is in general not the terrain of arresting cases involving heroic decisions or extraordinary circumstances arising at the extremes of medical practice; indeed, this may be one reason for the relative lack of attention it has attracted. Rather, it is the field of day-to-day communication and structured, complex interactions, of subtle gestures and fine nuances of language. Let us take another mundane example, this time of an elderly man who is anxiously awaiting the result of a biopsy of an abdominal mass that will show that he has metastatic cancer. How should the biopsy information be conveyed to him? Here, the patient will invest every gesture and every intonation of the voice of the physician with weighty implications. The event itself will live with him, and during the course of his illness he will often return to it in his memory; no subsequent medical intervention will have such a powerful impact or such enduring consequences. The quality of his life, what remains of it, and the decisions that he will make may well be determined at this time. The beginning of the conversation is straightforward enough: the doctor must make an opening statement and await the response of the patient; he must then provide the latter with an opportunity to consider the information and to determine what else he wants to know, or wants to avoid knowing. What happens after this cannot be predicted: it will depend on the doctor, the patient and their interaction. Many issues will arise. In what manner should the prognosis of the illness be discussed, for example, in response to the patient's direct inquiry? What if no such inquiry is made? Should the subject be raised in any case? What should be said about the pain, the discomfort and the uncertainty that can now be awaited? How should the physician respond to the man's despair, or to his bravado, or to his forced attempts at joviality? In this brief consultation an almost unlimited array of microethical issues is raised, each of which may carry enduring implications for the patient.

The clinical engagement with experiences of life that do not, or should not, be identified with pathology raises special microethical issues: for example, puberty, sexuality, menopause, ageing and childbirth. Some of these will be discussed in detail below.[13] We consider here briefly the last of these.

There has been considerable discussion in recent years about the 'medicalisation' of childbirth in Western societies, according to which traditional, often community or family-based, approaches to pregnancy and childbirth have been progressively replaced by practices that emphasise technical interventions and outcomes.[14] Even within the perspective of the dominant culture, however, it is widely recognised that the nature of the experience of childbirth may have long-standing consequences for both parents and children. The attention and care paid to the preparation for the labour may be especially important; this may include detailed discussions about many aspects of the process and the parents', the doctor's and the midwives' preferences regarding various possible courses of action that might need to be considered. The physical circumstances of the labour and delivery, including the kind of lighting that is used and the aural environment, may also be important, as may be the facilities available for use during the labour. In the course of the labour itself, the kinds of medical assessment that should be carried out and the manner in which they are employed need to be carefully examined. The communication of the results of the physical examinations, advice or suggestions regarding the activity of the woman, including the positions she might adopt, and the contributions of a partner may be very sensitive issues with powerful consequences. The more narrowly 'medical' interventions also raise the possibility of an inappropriate, possibly inadvertent, exercise of power by medical personnel in circumstances where the woman and her partner may be especially vulnerable. How should they be explained to the labouring woman, in order to obtain her consent? How should they be carried out? The 'medical indications' for such procedures can be found in standard textbooks. However, the possible enduring effects of an insensitively executed medical intervention cannot: the consequences of the fractured intimacy of the moment, and of the invasion of a profound experience, heavy with meaning, by gowned and gloved technicians. The medical management of a labour and delivery, therefore, has a complex ethical substratum. Decisions made at this level, furthermore, may be of great importance for the outcomes; indeed, it is possible to say that, in some respects at least, their importance may exceed that of the narrowly defined technical results.

The full appreciation of the microethical richness of clinical practice cannot be conveyed by brief, formal descriptions or case summaries: indeed, such descriptions and summaries threaten exactly the same, facile oversimplification for which we are taking bioethics to task. The second part of this book contains a number of more detailed reflections on the rich complexities of the clinical lifeworld. However, I would like to consider one further example. A medical student working in the Emergency Department was helping out by suturing a laceration in the scalp of an elderly man who had been injured in a motor car accident. The student had stitched up similar wounds under supervision several times in the past and was clearly competent to do so. During the course of the procedure it became apparent to her that the patient had assumed that she was a qualified doctor and expressed his confidence in her experienced manner. She felt uncomfortable with this misconception but was reluctant to enter into a detailed explanation of the true situation at such a sensitive moment. Accordingly, she decided not to disabuse him and to continue the inadvertent deception, even after she had finished the job. Subsequently, trying to come to terms with her sense of guilt, she sought advice about how she should have responded.

In her interactions with the elderly man and the execution of the procedure itself, the student had sought to deport herself impeccably. Indeed, her presence in the Emergency Department late on a Saturday night was itself a mark of her personal commitment and dedication. The contretemps in which she found herself immersed, however, left her deeply troubled and wondering whether she had betrayed the patient's trust and maybe discredited both herself and her colleagues.

It is easy to recognise here that telling a lie is wrong and to emphasise the importance of 'informed consent'. However, this may cover only part of the problem. As Eric Cassell has pointed out in an insightful commentary on a related case, ethical issues such as truth-telling do not stand alone as timeless principles: they are important only 'because of their place in human relations—of persons to themselves and to others'. Both the student and the patient are likely to be frightened and unsure; for this reason—and others—rather than being regarded as adversaries the two should be seen as natural allies. Both have much to gain from the interaction and, indeed, the experience may be enriched by the student's openness and readiness to learn. The latter must set out actively to win the trust of the patient and to justify that trust with her actions. She will then come to understand that the medical interaction is a mutual one. There are often doubts and uncertainties, for 'that is the nature of medical care', of the 'complex system of relationships and bonds that are part of the moral nature of the institution of medicine'.[15] This case shows, therefore, how the established ethical categories may be revealed as partial and inadequate and how much broader and richer the microethical issues are—and truer to the reality of clinical practice.

The domain of ethical issues in medicine is much larger and more diverse than is generally accepted within the paradigms of conventional bioethics. What is often omitted by the latter is precisely an appreciation of the microethical context of clinical medicine and of the crucial role of this context in medical decision-making. Although microethics may be more important for the determination of medical outcomes than most other factors, it is generally not considered in debates about medical ethics.

The consequences of this neglect of the microethical context of clinical medicine are substantial. Without an appreciation of the underlying structure of the reverberating physician–patient interaction, the nature of the medical relationship itself is obscured. The ethical decision-making process involving patient and doctor becomes profoundly distorted, seeming to be merely a matter of choosing, more or less arbitrarily, between alternatives rarely located in the real context of practical medicine and continuing interpersonal interaction. Communication between the participants becomes distorted, or is never truly begun; this, in turn, leads to an exaggerated dependence on formal legal 'solutions' to problems that ought to be resolved locally. In the worst cases, it leads to the dismembering of clinical practice itself, with the responsibility for many qualitative judgements being passed to committees or, worse, to individuals who claim expertise not in a delimited area of knowledge, but in one ('bioethical') component of the complex, intricate process of medical decision-making.

It should be clear how the microethical project differs from the bioethical one. Microethics starts from the premise that clinical practice consists of an accumulation of barely discernable ethical events. Accordingly, its task is to chart the topography of the medical lifeworld, as it exists in its concreteness, its fluidity and its temporal unpredictability. By this means, microethics seeks to reveal the structure and the dynamics of the clinical interaction and, in particular, to explicate the actual processes involved in clinical decision-making. The bioethical formulation of the ethical content of medicine is quite different. It focuses on formal descriptions of dilemmas, which are themselves derived by a process of abstraction from the practical discursive context. These dilemmas, then, are representations of clinical practice within a pre-given theoretical framework; to these representations, the methods and techniques of the theoretical system are subsequently applied.

Bioethics and microethics differ, therefore, both in epistemological terms and at the foundational level of the constitution of their objects. From the point of view of microethics, bioethics is not false, or erroneous, in the sense of contradicting the facts. Rather, it is considered to exist at a different level of generality and to be addressing different theoretical tasks. It is not a concern of bioethics to seek to apprehend in detail the complexity of the medical quotidian, and, indeed, it is not capable of doing so. Conversely, microethics is not concerned primarily with the formal structure of ethical dilemmas, which it considers to be of limited relevance for actual clinical practice. It does not deny, of course, as has been stated before, that dilemmas do occur from time to time in real practice and that classical bioethical considerations may then to a degree be useful. However, it contends that, in these very cases, the occurrence of a dilemma in itself is often merely indicative of a deeper problem—namely, the breakdown of the communicative process between the participants—so that in these circumstances this ought to become the main issue. In any event, regardless of the formulation, a 'microethical' solution—that is, one at the level of the actual interaction between doctor and patient—must ultimately always be found, so there is no means by which the microethical realisation of discourse can be circumvented.

The Clinic as the Foundation of Modern Medicine

Ethics is at the heart of medical practice. The face-to-face engagement of carer and sufferer is at the heart of the ethical life of the clinic. What is the position of microethics in relation to the other forms of discourse and action that constitute modern medicine? We need to clarify this status in order to define the ethical parameters in more detail and so to guide actual choices. Such a clarification is also useful in other respects, in that it allows certain theoretical problems of medicine—concerning both structural issues and questions of knowledge—to be elucidated.

Microethics is founded on the clinical experience itself, or more specifically in the communicative processes that emerge from the forms of interaction that characterise the medical relationship, in association with the wider community within which they are articulated. I will not attempt to provide a formal description of this theoretical foundation; it is much better to illustrate the fullness, the scope and the richness of the microethical domain through discussion of actual experiences, and this is what I will do in the second part of this book. Here, I will, however, make a few additional rudimentary remarks, in order to indicate some of the diverse resources on which a theory of microethics can call and so to establish lines of continuity between microethics and existing projects, to sketch some preliminary conclusions from the present deliberations, and to identify some problems for future consideration.

Social relationships in general do not occur independently of each other, nor do they subsist in isolation from other forms of social life. Every relationship exists within a system of discourse that circumscribes its communicative possibilities and sets out rules of behaviour. In other words, social life is partitioned into intersecting regions, or 'language games' (to use a term introduced by Wittgenstein) that form integrated systems of discourse and action. Each of these regions has its own structure, which determines its characteristic modes of communication and the associated forms of social action. The medical relationship supports a range of language games, each of which has its own particular structures that can be described in more or less precise detail. It carries a special interest because of the central role it plays within clinical medicine in general.

The medical interaction has a complex and dynamic structure, which develops from a number of disparate sources. The description of this structure is as yet incomplete. We are able to say, however, that there are several levels that are of importance. There is, first of all, what might be called a level of universal structural determinants. This embraces the structures that are common to all instances of communication and their associated normative imperatives. These have been studied under the general heading of 'universal pragmatics' or, more specifically, 'discourse ethics', by Karl-Otto Apel and Jürgen Habermas.[16] It also encompasses the historically determined central and formative role of the clinic in modern medicine, which has been described in detail by Michel Foucault and others, who have emphasised the importance of the changing nature of the relationship between doctor and patient in the history of medicine. The modern clinic, it must be said at once, is not a homogeneous entity; it has a complex structure that has yet to be fully elaborated.

At the highest possible level of generality, any interaction that has ethical content must take for granted certain assumptions—for example, about the nature of communication, about the rules of argumentation and about the possibility that the various participants will change their attitudes or beliefs as a direct result of the interchange itself. If these presuppositions cannot be vindicated in real-life situations, moral judgements or behaviour will no longer be possible. Apel and Habermas set themselves the task of explicating the logical structure of this ethical substratum of all communicative interactions. Utilising the strategy of a phenomenological description of the moral domain, they have sought to uncover the normative premises implicit in the acts that characterise the process of communication itself. The project is explicitly a Kantian one, in that its concern is with the transcendental conditions of possibility of discourse, or even of 'normativity'—indeed, the 'principle of universalisation' that emerges from it bears a clear and explicit relationship to the categorical imperative.[17] Nonetheless, it does make a substantial new departure, to the extent that it shifts the focus of ethical reflection back to the social and intersubjective engagements that constitute communicative processes.

There can be no doubt that at the basis of every medical interaction there are certain fundamental assumptions about social behaviour and ethical intercourse; furthermore, these undoubtedly are of great importance for the derivation of rules of ethical conduct within medicine. However—and this is readily accepted by Habermas[18]—these assumptions manifest themselves only in relation to the specific conditions of the particular practical discourse that characterises medicine. Similarly, universal, transcendentally grounded rules of conduct within medicine become meaningful there only when considered in relation to the real horizon of the medical lifeworld. For this reason, the identification of these rules and structures is intimately linked to the explication of the characteristic discursive landscape of the clinical encounter.

It is now well recognised that the advent of modern medicine consisted largely of the formation of the clinic—or, more precisely, the development of the clinical encounter—as the practical locus of both knowledge and action.[19] Pre-modern medicine relied on a variety of therapeutic and interpretative techniques derived from a number of sources, which were only loosely and informally related to the physician–patient interaction and lacked a basis in a rigorous theory of the body. The development of the clinic introduced a set of highly disciplined procedures for both observing the body and obtaining information. Of course, there were very complex conceptual transformations presupposed in the development and refinement of this 'clinical gaze'. Furthermore, the clinic itself assumed an ambivalence that has ever since been both productive and limiting: on the one hand, there was the 'scientific' reduction of disease and physical processes, which enabled the body to be opened up to systematic, empirical investigation; on the other, there was the ancient appreciation of the delicacy and mystery of embodied subjectivity and of the altered forms it assumes under conditions of illness. The former aspect derives, in the modern period, from the writings of Claude Bernard and his followers and has received much of the attention of historians of medicine (including Foucault). The latter can be traced back to the Hippocratic corpus; it has perdured alongside, and sometimes in opposition to, the scientific view. Its intellectual resources are different: within the clinical literature, Thomas Sydenham may be regarded as a notable advocate[20]; in contemporary times, the theory of embodiment has been developed in detail by a number of authors.[21]

The two great themes of the scientific and the existential accounts of disease stand together in the contemporary clinic in an uneasy tension. Indeed, this tension has become one of the distinguishing marks of modern medicine and is the source both of its extraordinary heterogeneity and the unquenchable public fascination it arouses. Of greater relevance for our present purposes than the difference between these two aspects, however, is the common ground they share, which has made some compromise between them possible. Both recognise the special role of the clinic; that is, the potential potency of the interaction between patient and doctor, sufferer and skilled interpreter. As different as their premises are, both perspectives accept that this relationship is the principle source of medical knowledge of disease and disease processes. Accordingly, for both, the clinical encounter is not just a forum for the exchange of information between two individuals. It is a sophisticated epistemological tool that enables all the potential sources of knowledge about the patient and his or her illness to be effectively mobilised: within it, as the structured, theoretical representation of the illness known as the 'history', the special knowledge of the patient is at last formally recognised and granted a legitimate status. This is placed alongside the knowledge deriving from the direct experience of the physician, now formalised into the 'physical examination'.[22]

The clinical encounter is a place where things are created and accomplished. It is where the implications of knowledge are tested and where therapeutic action is initiated and pursued. It has become the occasion where practical decisions are realised and subsequently adjusted, in the light both of their real outcomes and of the particular perspectives and value systems of the participating individuals.[23]

The relations between doctors and patients, therefore, emerge from the history of medicine as embracing highly refined systems of discourse closely linked to specific forms of action. Like other such systems that constitute the remainder of social life, these ones have pre-given internal structures and are linked to accompanying sets of behavioural injunctions. These injunctions may in turn reflect, at least in part, the universal conditions of communicative interactions, as they manifest themselves through the particular, concrete forms of the clinic. They impose, from within, a boundary on any given interaction; that is, the clinical interaction not only has internal structures but is also governed by internal limits.

The Uncontainable Openness of the Clinical Encounter

The universal constraints are by no means the only ones to which the doctor–patient relationship is subjected. There is another, critically important, set of structural determinants: the value systems of the individuals involved. On the face of it, this seems straightforward: simply, each person enters the medical encounter with a given, pre-existing set of values and value preferences. In reality, however, the advent of such systems of values is itself an extremely complex and difficult matter. This process has been studied in some detail[24]; in the present context it is sufficient to note merely that values are neither completely arbitrary nor fully determined. They are contingent on local traditions, on large-scale cultural allegiances and on the specific life circumstances of individuals, and they are subject to constraints linked to the social settings within which they are to be realised. They are themselves the outcomes of decisions and choices. While choices need to be made, in the modern world the range of available possibilities is very great: indeed, probably qualitatively greater than in any previous epoch.[25]

Once a relationship has been established, there is a need for an ongoing process of decision-making regarding various aspects of its conduct. These decisions will be subject to both the internal constraints (including personal values) and the external ones (the social milieu) we have mentioned. With respect to the medical encounter, it can be seen that the internal structure of the interaction itself and its implicit rules of conduct go a long way towards organising it in a functional sense. At the same time, the values of each participant further limit the realisation of the institutional structures. The medical interaction, therefore, as we have mentioned before, has a complex and heterogeneous structure; it is precisely this complex structure that generates the microethical imperatives.

The modern person—in Western, and increasingly in 'developing', societies—occupies many roles; more precisely, he or she participates in many of these systems of discourse and action, or language games. For example, a physician may also be a citizen, research worker, father or mother, teacher, or political activist. The assemblage of such language games together shape the totality of the meanings to which an individual's social interactions and personal commitments give rise. Individually, they delimit various regions of social life and shape particular types of behaviour and relationships.[26]

Language games may be highly heterogeneous, to the point that the goals and values potentially realisable within different settings may be in open conflict. Every person, however, learns to operate within the constraints of each relevant sphere of activity; that is, to follow the rules and to acquire facility with a variety of discourse systems. In each sphere, furthermore, decisions about right conduct need to be made. The demands of some may be different from those of others, as we have said. In addition, they may vary according to changing circumstances and, in particular, according to the ongoing interactions between subjects engaged in structured communication and dialogue within them.[27]

Interchanges between doctors and patients are extremely heterogeneous. They are subject to formal discursive regularities; that is, constant structural features of the clinical encounter that distinguish it from other interactions. However, at the same time, there is often quite unpredictable variation, related in part to the fact that both patients and health practitioners belong simultaneously to several—sometimes many—domains of activity, each of which has its own rules of conduct and its own more or less complex forms of communication and knowledge. To adopt the point of view of a doctor in a developed Western country, for the sake of illustration, in addition to his or her own highly variable roles, within the clinical encounter such a practitioner may be called upon to interact with many different kinds of people, each of whom has a distinctive set of values and goals. For example, it may not be surprising for a general practitioner working in the suburbs of Melbourne, Chicago or Paris in a single afternoon to see a young, gay professional man, a middle-aged female migrant factory worker and an elderly retired farmer who has taken the day off work to make the trip from the country. This range of interactions indicates the versatility that is demanded of practising clinicians in these cultural settings: they are required to be engaged in constant processes of transcription and translation across systems of discourse. The processes of communication must be adaptable to the needs of particular patients; what happens when mistakes are made at this level is very familiar.

The multiplicity and heterogeneity of language games reflects the pluralist nature of modern Western society. The proliferation of styles of communication and spheres of action is both liberating and limiting. It provides greatly expanded contexts for action. At the same, however, it imposes new constraints. This complexity may from time to time lead to the possibility of conflict between contending ethical duties and obligations.

******

The complex, multifaceted nature of the medical interaction is accessible to investigation with the help of a variety of well-established tools. These enable the structures of the medical lifeworld to be elucidated without loss of concreteness or specificity. The task is in part that of a phenomenological description of the experience of the clinic; however, it is not merely this, for it also requires an explication of relationships that are structured and laden with ethical imperatives. The medical lifeworld is multifaceted and highly differentiated; it contains among its irreducible elements forms of intersubjectivity that are historically structured. Superimposed on the universal structures are historically and socially contingent variables.

These considerations lead to a strong conclusion regarding medical relationships that has profound implications for ethical decision-making. The interactions that occur in the medical encounter and the decisions that come out of them are largely unpredictable, just as are the value systems that are superimposed upon them. They depend very sensitively not only on the precise factual details of the patient's illness but also on the courses of the actual interchanges that occur between patients and physicians.[28] Accordingly, the relationships are, from the outset, indeterminate; that is, the cumulative outcome of a series of decisions may be very different from a decision that might seem to be preferred in retrospect, with full knowledge of all of the circumstances that subsequently developed. Every clinician is familiar with this phenomenon, which is illustrated in some of the cases in the second part of this book: the result of a long series of decisions, each of which has been taken in good faith and after careful consideration, may be the very outcome that at the beginning seemed least desirable.

There are no 'typical cases' in clinical medicine from the point of view of ethics or communicative dialogue. Each 'case' has its own irreducible particularity. Both parties enter the relationship with values and expectations, but without knowing what will be discovered and what will thus be created. This fundamental conclusion vitiates a large part of the contemporary discourse about 'medical ethics'; it means also that there is no alternative to the microethical route.

Another example may be helpful here, which illustrates both the nature of clinical practice and the inadequacy of the bioethical perspective. The question is occasionally posed in ethics classes for medical students about what they would do if a patient of theirs were diagnosed as having a serious sexually transmitted disease and they were later to learn that he or she was about to start a relationship with a personal friend of the student. At first glance, the problem seems straightforward: it invites the students to consider whether they would favour releasing confidential information to a third person and the expected debate would be concerned with the value of confidentiality and its limitations, especially in relation to the principles of autonomy, non-maleficence, beneficence and justice, and possibly with the legal implications of both disclosure and non-disclosure.[29]

In the real situation, however, as students themselves invariably realise, what occurs is something very different. A process of discussion is initiated between the doctor and the patient and there is a parallel process of personal reflection for each. It is possible that the discussion will continue for some time as the patient comes to terms with his or her anger or bewilderment at the fact of the diagnosis and each party works through a range of complex feelings relating to responsibility, contending loyalties, guilt and maybe other issues. Where the debate ends no-one can say—and indeed, no-one ought to be able to say, if human interactions are to retain meaningful content. An infinite array of outcomes is possible; some of these have desirable and some have undesirable implications. The question that is suggested in the bioethical formulation may not ultimately be the most important issue, or, indeed, it may even turn out not to be an issue at all: in fact, it is extremely uncommon for a patient to refuse to tell a friend or relative about a possible medical risk. Instead, what may emerge as most important may be, for example, the patient's own concerns about his or her body; it may be the fear of illness or even death; it may be anxiety about a particular relationship or about relationships in general; or it may involve concern about apparently extraneous matters like employment or financial security. These considerations may seem to be begging the question of ethical debate; nonetheless, they are precisely the ones that predominate in clinical work. In clinical interactions, all we can do is to say where we will start and how we will proceed; the rest is—subject to the requirements of microethical structures—up to the interchange itself.

******

In this chapter, I have been discussing the practical business of medical decision-making. I have highlighted the estrangement of much of contemporary ethical discourse from the real experiences of the clinic and its inability to provide the insights and guidance required to respond to the concerns of the community about the way in which medicine has developed. Approaches to ethics that share a common root with the technical commitment of medicine do not have access to domains of meaning that lie outside science and, as a result, a large component of the deep experience with which medicine deals is invisible to them.

I have argued that in the flow of the clinical interaction, a continuum of decisions of almost infinitesimal magnitude arises. Each of these decisions has a small but finite ethical content; their cumulative sum determines both the qualitative and the quantitative outcomes of the medical encounter. Clinical practice proceeds by such local, piecemeal mechanisms. At the outset of most clinical relationships, the overall outcomes are largely indeterminate.

These results are basic facts of modern medicine that must be accepted by anyone—doctor or patient—who participates in it. The microethical aspect of medicine is not merely incidental. It is of central importance both for clinical practice and for the understanding of what medicine can and cannot do. It is part of the living core of clinical practice.

Notes

1 See, for example: I Illich, *Limits to Medicine* (London, Marion Boyars, 1976); R Taylor, *Medicine Out of Control* (Melbourne, Sun Books, 1979); G Corea, *The Mother Machine. From Artificial Insemination to Artificial Wombs* (New York, Harper & Row, 1985).
2 RL Holmes, 'The Limited Relevance of Analytical Ethics to the Problems of Bioethics', *Journal of Medicine and Philosophy*, 15(2), 1990: 143–60; BA Brody, 'Quality of Scholarship in Bioethics', *Journal of Medicine and Philosophy*, 15(2), 1990: 161–78.
3 CM Culver, *Ethics at the Bedside* (Dartmouth, University Press of New England, 1990); M Siegler, 'Clinical Ethics and Clinical Medicine', *Archives of Internal Medicine*, 139, 1979: 914–5; CD Clements, 'Bioethical Essentialism and Scientific Population Thinking', *Perspectives in Biology and Medicine*, 28(2), 1985: 188–207; EJ Cassell, *The Healer's Art: A New Approach to the Doctor–Patient Relationship* (Philadelphia, J.B. Lipincott, 1976).
4 RM Zaner, *Ethics and the Clinical Encounter* (Edgeworth Cliffs, NJ, Prentice-Hall, 1988); A Frank, *At the Will of the Body: Reflections on Illness* (Boston, Houghton Mifflin Co., 1991); RC Fox, 'Evolution of American Bioethics: A Sociological Perspective', in G Weisz, ed., *Social Science Perspectives on Medical Ethics* (Netherlands, Kluwer, 1990), pp. 201–17; C Elliott, *A Philosophical Disease: Bioethics, Culture, and Identity* (New York, Routledge, 1999); LA Eckenwiler and FG Cohn, eds, *The Ethics of Bioethics: Mapping the Moral Landscape* (Baltimore, Johns Hopkins University Press, 2007); S Fish, *The Trouble with Principle* (London, Harvard University Press, 1999).
5 A MacIntyre, *After Virtue: A Study in Moral Theory* (London, Duckworth, 1987); B Williams, *Ethics and the Limits of Philosophy* (London, Fontana, 1985); C Taylor, *Sources of the Self: The Making of the Modern Identity* (Cambridge, Harvard University Press, 1989); see also M Charlesworth, 'Bioethics and the Limits of Philosophy', *Bioethics News*, 9(1), 1989: 1–24;

C Gilligan, *In a Different Voice: Psychological Theory and Women's Development* (London, Harvard University Press, 1982).

6 See M Siegler, 'Clinical Ethics and Clinical Medicine'; cf. also C Elliott, *A Philosophical Disease*, and LA Eckenwiler and FG Cohn, *The Ethics of Bioethics*.

7 See, for example: TL Beauchamp JF and Childress, *Principles of Biomedical Ethics* (Oxford University Press, 1983); TL Beauchamp and L Walters, eds, *Contemporary Issues in Bioethics* (Belmont, CA, Wadsworth Publishing Company, 1982); RM Veatch, *A Theory of Medical Ethics* (New York, Basic Books, 1981); J Glover, *Causing Death and Saving Lives* (New York, Penguin Books, 1977); P Singer, *Practical Ethics* (Cambridge University Press, 1979); TL Regan, ed., *Matters of Life and Death. New Introductory Essays in Moral Philosophy* (New York, Random House, 1980).

8 ED Pellegrino and DC Thomasma, *A Philosophical Basis of Medical Practice* (New York, Oxford University Press, 1981); O O'Neill, *Autonomy and Trust in Bioethics* (Cambridge, Cambridge University Press, 2002); RM Zaner, *Ethics and the Clinical Encounter*; D Crane, *The Sanctity of Social Life: Physicians' Treatment of Critically Ill Patients* (New York, Russell Sage, 1975); J Ladd, 'The Internal Morality of Medicine: An Essential Dimension of the Patient–Physician Relationship', in EA Shelp, ed., *The Clinical Encounter: The Moral Fabric of the Physician–Patient Relationship* (Dordrecht, Reidel, 1983), pp. 209–31.

9 The major reports that have considered in detail the questions associated with ethics teaching in medical courses have not considered the microethical issues. See PA Komesaroff, 'The Nature of Medicine and the Teaching of Medical Ethics', *Bioethics*, 4(1), 1990: 66–77.

10 cf. EJ Cassell, *Talking with Patients* (Cambridge, MA, MIT Press, 1985).

11 cf. J La Puma and DL Schiedermayer, 'The Clinical Ethicist at the Bedside', *Theoretical Medicine*, 12, 1991: 141–9; and DS Davis, 'Rich Cases: The Ethics of Thick Description', *Hastings Centre Report*, 21(4), 1991: 12–16. See also CM Culver, *Ethics at the Bedside*.

12 Although, as mentioned, evidence for the clinical utility of bioethics is lacking, in relation to the microethical variables, such evidence abounds. For example, one method of studying the outcomes of clinical medicine is to examine 'patient satisfaction'; here, the evidence points strongly in favour of microethics. See, for example, JA Hall and MC Dornan, 'What Patients Like about Their Medical Care and How Often They Are Asked: A Meta-analysis of the Satisfaction Literature', *Soc Sci Med*, 27(9), 1988: 935–9; BS Hulka, LL Kupper, JC Cassel and RA Babineau, 'Practice Characteristics and Quality of Primary Medical Care: The Doctor–Patient Relationship', *Medical Care*, 13(10), 1975: 808–20.

13 See especially Chapters 4 and 5.

14 See, for example, I Illich, *Limits to Medicine*, and G Corea, *The Mother Machine*.

15 For additional examples, see RM Zaner, *Ethics and the Clinical Encounter*, and EJ Cassell, *Talking with Patients*.

16 See, for example, J Habermas, *Moral Consciousness and Communicative Action* (Cambridge, MA, MIT Press, 1990); K-O Apel, *Towards the Transformation of Philosophy* (London, Routledge and Kegan Paul, 1980); S Benhabib and F Dallmayr, eds, *The Communicative Ethics Controversy* (Cambridge, MA, MIT, 1990); D Rasmussen, ed., *Universalism vs. Communitarianism: Contemporary Debates in Ethics* (Cambridge, MA, MIT, 1990).
17 J Habermas, 'Discourse Ethics: Notes on a Programme of Philosophical Justification', in S Benhabib and F Dallmayr, *The Communicative Ethics Controversy*, p. 90.
18 ibid., pp. 100–1.
19 M Foucault, *The Birth of the Clinic* (London, Tavistock, 1973). See also EJ Pellegrino and DC Thomasma, *A Philosophical Basis of Medical Practice*; EJ Pellegrino, 'The Healing Relationship: The Architechtonics of Clinical Medicine', in EA Shelp, *The Clinical Encounter*, pp. 153–72; MC Rawlinson, 'Foucault's Strategy: Knowledge, Power and the Specificity of Truth', *J Med Phil*, 12, 1987: 371–96.
20 It is claimed by T Engelhardt that, by '(bracketing) philosophical and scientific presuppositions' in order to 'describe the presented reality of patient's illnesses', Sydenham sought to develop 'an eidetic phenomenology of disease'. See HT Engelhardt, Jr, 'Illnesses, Diseases and Sicknesses', in V Kestenbaum, ed., *The Humanity of the Ill. Phenomenological Perspectives* (Knoxville, Tennessee, University of Tennessee Press, 1982), pp. 142–57.
21 See M Merleau-Ponty, *The Phenomenology of Perception* (London, Routledge and Kegan Paul, 1960); P Ricoeur, *Freedom and Nature: The Voluntary and the Voluntary* (Evanston, North-western University Press, 1966). See also RM Zaner, *The Problem of Embodiment* (The Hague, Martinus Nijhoff, 1971); RM Zaner, 'Embodiment', in WT Reich, *The Encyclopedia of Bioethics* (London, Free Press, 1978), pp. 361–6; D Leeder, 'Medicine and Paradigms of Embodiment', *J Med Phil*, 9(1), 1984: 29–44; MC Rawlinson, 'Medicine's Discourse and the Practice of Medicine', in V Kestenbaum, *The Humanity of the Ill*, pp. 69–85.
22 cf. G Canguilhem, *On the Normal and the Pathological* (Dordrecht, D. Reidel, 1978).
23 See V Kestenbaum, ed., 'Introduction: The Experience of Illness', in V Kestenbaum, *The Humanity of the Ill*, pp. 3–39, and other essays in this volume; and RM Zaner, *The Context of Self* (Ohio University Press, 1981).
24 L Kohlberg, *The Philosophy of Moral Development: Moral Stages and the Idea of Justice* (San Francisco, Harper & Row, 1981); J Piaget, *The Moral Judgement of the Child* (London, Routledge and Kegan Paul, 1965); J Habermas, *Moral Consciousness and Communicative Action*. See also C Gilligan, *In a Different Voice*.
25 A Heller, *A Philosophy of Morals* (London, Blackwell, 1990), chapters 1, 4.
26 L Wittgenstein, *Philosophical Investigations*, tr. GEM Anscombe (Oxford, Basil Blackwell, 1974); K-O Apel, *Towards the Transformation of Philosophy*, chapter 1; cf. also R Sokolowski, 'The Art and Science of

Medicine', in ED Pellegrino, JP Langan and JC Harvey, eds, *Catholic Perspectives on Medical Morals: Foundational Issues* (Boston, Kluwer Academic, 1989), pp. 263–75. Other formulations of related ideas may be found in the works of other authors; for example, 'finite provinces of meaning' (Schutz) or 'social practices' (MacIntyre). The concept of 'language game' is also employed—albeit with a somewhat different content—by J-F Lyotard in *The Postmodern Condition: A Report on Knowledge* (Manchester, Manchester University Press, 1986).

27 See also G Skirbekk, 'Contextual and Universal Pragmatics: Mutual Criticism of Praxeological and Transcendental Pragmatics', *Thesis 11*, 28, 1991: 35–51; and R Sokolowski, 'The Art and Science of Medicine', pp. 263–75.

28 cf. M Weber, 'Politics as a Vocation', in HH Gerth and CW Mills, eds, *From Max Weber* (London, Routledge and Kegan Paul, 1948), pp. 77–128; RM Zaner, *Ethics and the Clinical Encounter*, chapter 1.

29 See, for example, L Walters, 'Ethical Aspects of Medical Confidentiality', in TL Beauchamp and L Walters, eds, *Contemporary Issues in Bioethics* (California, Wadsworth Publishing Co., 1978), pp. 169–75; R Gillon, 'AIDS and Medical Confidentiality', *Brit Med J*, 294, 1987: 1675–7; A Orr, 'Legal AIDS: Implications of AIDS for British and American Law', *J Med Eth*, 15, 1989: 161–7.

CHAPTER 3
Between Nature and Culture
The Ethics and Politics of Animal Experimentation

Every year, vast numbers of non-human animals are used in scientific research; in the United States alone it is estimated that the total may reach 100 million.[1] Some of these are subjected to stressful or painful experiences as part of the experiments in which they are employed; most are killed at the end. Much of the study of disease, the search for new therapeutic agents in medicine and biological research in general, depends on animal studies. Many important discoveries have been made as a direct result of animal experimentation and many important therapeutic innovations have been made possible; examples include the discovery of antibiotics and of drugs for the treatment of pain, inflammatory disorders and cardiac and renal diseases; the development of many vaccines, including those against polio, measles and hepatitis; the discovery of insulin and its use in the treatment of diabetes; and the development of many new surgical techniques. In addition, animal research supports a substantial industry that provides livelihoods for the many people involved in the production and care of the animals, not to mention the livelihoods of the scientific workers themselves.

Opposition to animal experimentation has existed—in various forms and degrees of intensity—for many years. In the last decade or so in particular, however, it has developed into a powerful movement with wide support in many countries. As a result, the scientific community, which was at first inclined to dismiss the concern about the nature of its work as no more than a temporary aberration contrived by a few extremists, now finds itself faced with a coalition of philosophers, political activists and interested citizens commanding an international organisational network. The 'animal liberation' movement, or, more correctly, movements, furthermore have not been without influence on governments; indeed, in many countries there now exists an array of regulations and restrictions on scientific work that only a few years ago would have seemed inconceivable and that in some areas now actually threatens the possibility of ongoing research. In some instances, opponents of animal experimentation have resorted to violence: laboratories have been ransacked, experiments have been destroyed or damaged and scientists subjected to personal harassment, death threats to themselves or family members and in some cases physical violence.

It is widely recognised that during this process, scientists as a group have not defended themselves very effectively. This is in itself remarkable, given the high public profile of science and the ready accessibility of the mass media to the scientific community. It has been claimed that the success of the anti-vivisection movement has been due to an unwillingness on the part of the experimenters to communicate their cause publicly. The reality, however, is not so simple. The fact that scientists find themselves on the defensive has been due not so much to insufficient attention to public relations as to a failure to appreciate the depth and importance of the whole animal liberation phenomenon. Scientists have assumed that the public interest requires animal experimentation; as a result, they have largely refused to consider seriously the arguments put forward by those who oppose them. With a few notable exceptions, they have not attempted to understand what has become a significant social movement and, therefore, the insights that it can offer have remained inaccessible to them.

This chapter is an attempt to look again at the animal experimentation controversy with a view to redressing this deficiency, at least in part. It does not in any way pretend to offer a resolution to the disputes; indeed, it does not even take a position on the question of the morality of animal experimentation itself. Rather, the concern is with the philosophical and social roots of the contemporary opposition to the use of animals in science and, especially, with the kinds of discourse that have been employed by the various parties to the debate. One of the most remarkable features of the entire controversy has been the peculiar lack of communication between the two sides; this is especially noteworthy since the philosophical starting points of all the major contributors are very similar. This in itself is of considerable importance and, accordingly, particular attention will be directed to it.

Before proceeding, a word about terminology is needed. In this chapter, the terms 'anti-vivisectionists' and 'animal liberation movement' will be used broadly to include the diverse groups and individuals opposed to animal experimentation. 'Scientist' will be used as an abbreviation to refer to those members of the scientific community who either participate directly or acquiesce in experimentation involving non-human animals. The expression 'animals' will be employed to refer primarily to non-human animals. Finally, 'experimentation' will refer exclusively to research for the purposes of obtaining new scientific knowledge. Other uses of animals that are sometimes regarded under the general heading of 'animal research'—including the testing of cosmetics and other household products—will not be considered: the justifications for these practices are distinct from those for scientific research and, indeed, scientists are among the many members of the community who publicly question them.

The Problem

Experimentation on animals in one form or another goes back at least to the time of Galen in the second century CE. However, the use of animals in a systematic way as a tool for research in the familiar sense is of relatively recent origin, having been introduced into scientific practice about the middle of the eighteenth century.[2]

By the early nineteenth century, the use of animals in research had become commonplace, especially in the United Kingdom. At around this time, opposition, which had previously been scanty and fragmented, became organised into a number of groups concerned to protect the 'welfare' of animals. In England, the most prominent of these was the Society for the Prevention of Cruelty to Animals, later to be the Royal Society; its main platform was vigorous opposition to what was considered to be the inhumane treatment of animals and, especially, to the practice of 'vivisection'. On many occasions, therefore, these groups came into conflict with scientists. However, as has been widely noted, this opposition did not in general extend to a critique of the basic assumptions held by the society regarding non-human animals, let alone those regarding science itself. In particular, the fundamental propositions on which animal experimentation was premised—the assumptions that humans had dominion over the animal world, and that intrinsically animals were ethically of less consequence than humans—were essentially never questioned.

At the height of their popularity, the various animal protection societies were able to boast many thousands of members. The social basis for the movement was not wide, being largely dependent on the middle classes. It nonetheless succeeded in obtaining some notable victories, the most important of which was the passing of the *Cruelty to Animals Act* by the English Parliament in 1876. This Act, for the first time, established in legislation stringent conditions for animal care in scientific research. As it happened, this particular moment of triumph also marked the zenith of the movement's strength, for subsequently both its membership and influence declined sharply. The reasons for this decline are still debated. However, it is certain that one contributing factor was the dogged insistence by the main protagonists that animal experimentation in general lacked scientific validity. This was a fatal argument on which to rest the movement's credibility, for, with the proliferation of scientific discoveries and medical advances linked directly to animal research, the case of the scientists quickly prevailed. Indeed, the movement's popularity became so badly eroded that it was not for another three-quarters of a century that animal researchers were to encounter widespread and effective opposition.

At first glance, it may appear that the contemporary movements against animal experimentation represent nothing more than a revival of the preoccupations—and, some would say, prejudices—of the old animal protection societies. This is, however, not at all the case. The contemporary movements in fact mark a new departure at the levels of both theory and culture. They have, indeed, placed on the social agenda fundamental questions that were hitherto neglected: questions about the nature of science and its relationship to society, about the distinction between human and animal and about the link between knowledge and ethics.

The animal liberation movement is a social phenomenon of importance and complexity, and it would thus be expected that the questions it raises might issue in vigorous and productive interchanges among the various protagonists. However, useful dialogue between the two sides has been a remarkably rare event. More commonly, strong statements of position and bitter accusations have taken the place of reasoned argument. To a certain extent this has no doubt been due to the intense feelings generated on each side: the anti-vivisectionists have often been strident and tendentious in their arguments, and the scientists dogmatic and inflexible. However, the lack of communication goes deeper than this and must be regarded as a symptom of more fundamental issues. This chapter sets out to demonstrate that there are in fact important structural reasons within the bioethical discourse why the scientists and the anti-vivisectionists seem so often to be talking at cross-purposes, and that these reasons need to be elucidated if we are to discover what the two sides have to learn from each other; in other words, both the form and the contents of the arguments on both sides must be analysed if communication is to be restored. To commence this task, it is natural to start with a brief resume of the main positions adopted by the various protagonists.

Opposing Views

Both the scientists and the anti-vivisectionists usually formulate their arguments in the language of bioethical discourse. As we shall see, this is itself of interest because it fixes the theoretical parameters of the debate somewhat narrowly, excluding in particular the metatheoretical questions on the one hand, as well as the social and political ones on the other. In subsequent sections it will be argued that the debate about animal experimentation in fact throws into question some fundamental precepts about ethical analysis, as well as some basic concepts like 'environment', 'ecology' and even 'nature' itself.

The scientists and their supporters most commonly argue from a straightforward consequentialist point of view. Experimentation is good, so it is claimed, because of the beneficial consequences it produces for humans—and even, on occasions, for animals. This argument is certainly a strong one and, as we have noted, is based on secure factual evidence. This remains so despite occasional instances, well-documented by the animal liberationists, of irrelevant, unnecessary or badly devised experiments.[3]

As with consequentialist positions in general, the argument does not stand on its own; it needs to be supported by non-consequentialist propositions that justify the overall strategy of argumentation. In this case, the most important of these is the belief that from an ethical point of view, animals are inherently less valuable than human beings; this may be put slightly less strongly as the proposition that as a general principle, beneficial consequences for humans should outweigh harmful ones for animals. Where an attempt to further justify this distinction between humans and animals is made, it is usually on the basis of what are thought to be crucial differences between the two. This strategy has a very long history: Aristotle considered that animals were distinguished from humans by the absence among them of political organisation; Rousseau thought that the lack of free will was vital; the later thinkers of the Enlightenment located the crucial difference at the level of the inability of animals to reason, while Hegel felt that their lack of self-consciousness was decisive. Other philosophers have drawn attention to additional properties claimed to be characteristic of human beings that animals purportedly lack, such as language, social organisation, individual identity or the ability to anticipate the future.

Needless to say, both the relevance of these distinctions and their factual basis have been rigorously questioned. However, perhaps more interesting than this is the fact that despite the arguments, it is rare today for the extreme form of the 'human dominionism' position to be applied in practice—that is to say, it is rare for the view to be defended that animals have no moral standing, so that no amount of pain or suffering inflicted on them is of consequence. Instead, most scientists appear to feel intuitively that it is wrong to hurt animals if this can be avoided. As a result, voluntary codes of ethics are widely observed that prohibit cruel or painful experiments, or experiments for which the potential gains are not considered to justify the sacrifice of animal lives.

Other arguments are occasionally put forward to support animal experimentation. Of these, a particularly interesting one is the claim that knowledge itself is a sufficiently important value to justify animal experimentation in its own right, independently of specific consequences for either animals or humans. This view clearly has deep cultural roots and has been absorbed by science as part of its contemporary ideological justification. As we shall see later, this important assumption forms a dividing line between the two sides.

In their arguments, the anti-vivisectionists adopt various approaches.[4] However, essentially, all share a simple common theme. Animals, it is claimed, cannot be differentiated ethically on the basis of membership of a given species alone. It is conceded that there may be morally relevant differences between individuals that are linked to their physiological constitution, such as the ability to experience pain. It is argued, however, that even in these cases it is only the differences that are important ethically and not the physical data themselves.

According to the anti-vivisection perspective, once the 'speciesist' assumption has been dismissed, animal experimentation considered on its merits is seen to be generally wrong. From a utilitarian point of view, the argument is roughly as follows. Valid ethical comparisons involving individual animals of different species can be made only by considering the capacities of the various animals for experiencing pleasure or happiness, or pain and suffering. In cases where different kinds of animals share the same interests—as, for example, in relation to the avoidance of pain—the interests of all of them must be given equal weight. The application of this argument leads to the conclusion that in the vast majority of cases, the benefits obtained from research involving animals will be outweighed by the negative consequences for the animals themselves; in these cases the research must be judged to be morally wrong. It may be noted that while this argument would exclude most research involving animals, it does not prohibit it absolutely, since it is conceivable that in some cases the benefits would at least justify some animal suffering.

From a deontological perspective, the opposition to the use of animals in research is usually less compromising. Here, several possible arguments are employed. One viewpoint, for example, claims that animal experimentation is wrong in principle because, simply, it is wrong to kill or to inflict pain on a living thing. Another argument that has acquired contemporary popularity is that animals possess 'rights' that legally and morally should be considered to be of equal standing to those enjoyed by humans; these rights are necessarily infringed by animal experimentation, which therefore must be regarded as wrong. In both of these cases the argument is based on an underlying assumption, the justification of which derives from either the intuition of the individual or the prevailing legal and moral tradition.

It is not intended here to attempt to give a comprehensive account of the entire debate about animal experimentation; the aim, a more limited one, is to make three points. First, there are strong arguments available to each side, which indeed are commonly put forward cogently and articulately; this is evident and needs no further elaboration. Secondly, attention should be drawn to the fact that, despite their widely divergent and incompatible conclusions, both scientists and animal liberationists share certain basic assumptions and rely on a common intellectual tradition; this will be explained in some detail below. However, it is clear most obviously, for example, that each side not only feels the need to establish its particular case by means of ethical arguments, but that each also employs the same formal conditions for assessing the validity of an argument. Indeed, it is apparent that although the animal liberation argument was not articulated in full detail and rigour until relatively recently, in a theoretical sense it was always a formal possibility within the Western philosophical tradition; the reasons for the historical neglect of this viewpoint are themselves of interest and are yet to be fully explored.

Each side, then, can command powerful arguments and neither is obviously the stronger; certainly, there are no self-evident theoretical criteria that enable an uncommitted outsider to choose decisively between the two points of view. Importantly, however—and this is the third point—it is frequently the case that the opposing positions are not able to communicate effectively with each other. To be sure, failure of communication between different ethical points of view is not especially remarkable—the public debates about abortion provide an obvious additional example of the same phenomenon. The case of animal experimentation, however, is especially important because it raises fundamental issues regarding some of the deepest assumptions of our culture. The communication blockage that characterises the animal experimentation debate is in fact a symptom of deep social divisions and theoretical prejudices that are built into the very structure of bioethical discourse. Its elucidation will require a questioning of both science and ethics.

Science Versus Ethics

It is widely assumed—not just in the debates about animal experimentation—that ethics and science are independently constituted bodies of thought that intersect only incidentally at the periphery. It is true, as we shall see, that the two can be distinguished by means of a range of criteria. In spite of this, their relationship is a very intimate one: they are mutually dependent at a deep theoretical level as well as in terms of their social presuppositions and implications.

The distinction between science and ethics can be drawn in several ways. Perhaps the most obvious is in terms of the objects with which they deal: for science, the objects are those things that belong to 'nature'—comprising either physical or biological phenomena—while ethics deals with values, or, at least, with acts associated with values. Similarly, the processes of thought and of argument also differ fundamentally. The analytical logic of science and scientific thought is well characterised; the logic of ethical argument, by contrast, is both more heterogeneous and more variable, since it depends not just on formal rules of inference or deduction but also on the structures of communication and interaction. Thus, while it is unthinkable that contradictory propositions could be mutually true in science, in ethics, no law of the excluded middle applies: it is perfectly possible—and, indeed, a familiar occurrence—for two individuals, openly and in good faith, to hold opposing, and equally valid, ethical views. A third distinction related to this can be drawn in relation to the standards by which the validity of propositions is judged. For science, the criterion of validity is, of course, 'truth', which is assessed in various ways that have been widely discussed. For ethics, however, truth is not the issue; rather, the concern is primarily with what is 'right' or 'good'. A substantial literature over many centuries has addressed the distinction that is at issue here.

Another difference between ethics and science that is less convincing but also frequently asserted is that science is inscribed within what is referred to as the 'technical interest of knowledge'[5]—that is, that science by its very nature is committed to a mechanistic and objectivistic approach to its objects. Science, according to this view, is restricted to the analysis of causal processes (in the narrow sense of efficient causality alone) and its interventions are necessarily instrumental; the understanding of complex, organic unities is, according to this view, strictly outside the limits of science, as is an appreciation of the role of subjectivity and social interaction in the shaping of scientific propositions. Ethics, on the other hand, is said to occupy exactly the territory from which science is supposedly excluded: ethics inhabits the realms of society, of interaction and dialogue between individuals. There can be no doubt that, having regard to the most familiar forms of science, this characterisation carries a certain plausibility and in some contexts may even provide a useful framework for analysis. However, the underlying view of science that it promotes is profoundly misleading. The structures and processes of communication constitute the ineluctable substratum of not just ethics but of science as well.

Both science and ethics are, in fact, inherently social. This is not just in the obvious, 'weak' senses that the facts discovered by scientific investigation have social implications or imperatives and that nature itself is transformed by industry and the other effects of society that throw up new problems and possibilities for research. Rather, science and ethics are immanently social in a deeper and more far-reaching sense. Both are social accomplishments at the conceptual as well as the practical level: both depend on theoretical presuppositions that derive their meanings from particular social and historical configurations.

These arguments have been elaborated in detail elsewhere.[6] Here, it is sufficient to observe that the great innovations of Galileo, like those of Descartes, Diderot, D'Alembert, Bacon and others, were not primarily technical or mathematical in the narrow sense, but rather conceptual and philosophical, providing the philosophical prerequisites, the theoretical conditions of possibility, for the development of classical physics. These insights enabled the world to be restructured at a theoretical level in a manner that was not only accessible to physics but actually demanded its formulations. With the eighteenth-century European Enlightenment, the Galilean project of the interpretation of nature through the language of mathematics was systematically elaborated. Science became understood as a critical component of a social project, the goal of which was breathtakingly ambitious: to secure the liberation of mankind through the complete mastery and domination of both external and internal nature. For almost 200 years, this noble objective guided the aspirations of scientists, philosophers, social theorists and political movements.

The age of the Enlightenment was truly a time of the loss of innocence for Western thought. Its underlying project—of liberation through control and domination—was a political one, which guided and circumscribed the subsequent development not only of science and ethics but of society itself. The goal of science within this project, as we have said, was to master nature for the benefit of human society. This was a radically anthropocentric view that carried major consequences: now, human liberation and knowledge were the only standards according to which any phenomenon or act could be judged. Accordingly, non-human animals simply did not possess any inherent moral standing; indeed, for the thinkers of the Enlightenment, their moral status was no different from that of the inanimate objects of nature.[7]

Ethical thinking and its self-interpretation were brought under the same project. Despite their formal differences, both the overall goals of philosophical ethics and its theoretical objectives—as expressed through its methods of argument and analysis—became continuous with those of science. Ethics and freedom were now coterminous, for, as Diderot put it, 'if man is not free ... there can be no rational goodness or wickedness'. The goal of ethical thought, then, like that of science, was human liberation; accordingly, its standards were similarly anthropocentric. In addition, its theoretical objectives, again like those of science, included the abolition of doubt and the establishment of reliable locations for phenomena within systematic unities subject to irrefragable laws; after all—this time the words are those of Helvetius—if the physical universe is subject to the laws of motion, then the moral universe is equally subject to laws of its own. Thus, the great ethical systems of the time sought to provide simple, clear and definitive answers to these dilemmas, which had exercised and perplexed thinkers through the ages. Certainty, reproducibility and control became the objectives, if not the distinguishing marks, of both philosophical thought and the theory of nature.

Of course, not all the thinkers of the Enlightenment reached the same conclusions and not all adopted the same methods. The theory that represents most rigorously and completely a rational theory of ethical judgement was that developed by Immanuel Kant. However, as MacIntyre has shown[8], Kant's project of the rational justification of morality faithfully realised one of the most basic goals of Enlightenment thought, and in this respect represented a continuation of the projects of Diderot, Hume and others. The utilitarianism of the latter and the materialism of the former represent different solutions to a common problem. The fact that Hume was drawn to conclude—unlike Kant—that morals could not be derived from reason was less important than his abiding conviction that it remained subject to universal laws that could be elaborated, at least in part, in terms of a rational science of behaviour.

Science and ethics, despite their inherent differences, became intimately entwined under the banner of the Enlightenment. They came to serve the same social project and even deployed homologous theoretical structures. This proved to be simultaneously both a great strength and a fatal weakness. It was a strength not only because science was thereby endowed with an inherent ethical imprimatur, but also because the great power of scientific thought could now be mobilised in the interests of philosophical analysis. At the same time, however, it was a weakness, because it abolished the independent ground from which a critical reflection on science could be launched; the very fact that science and ethics now shared the same underlying goals and formal structures obviated any uncommitted philosophical analysis of either the techniques or the outcomes of science.

If these conclusions—presented here in only the most fragmentary form—are correct, then the ethical mode of analysis that emerged from the Enlightenment encountered an inexorable internal obstacle when it sought to turn its attention to the sciences of nature. As we shall see, the hegemony of this tradition of thought, with its deep anthropocentric biases, explains at least in part the uncritical attitude of most philosophical thought towards animal research. At the same time, it enables us to recognise the theoretical complexity and novelty of the contemporary anti-vivisection movement.

The question that arises concerns no less than the value that is placed on the objects of science; that is, the ethical standing of nature, or at least that part of it that comprises non-human animal life.

To consider the possibility of an ethical reflection on nature, it will be helpful to examine some aspects of the concept of nature itself, together with the related concepts of environment, ecology and ecological crisis.

Nature, Environment and Ecology

As we have seen, the objects with which science deals—that to which we refer collectively as 'nature'—are highly refined constructions that presuppose both social and conceptual antecedents. Although they are often taken for granted by working scientists as the primary and self-evident givens from which their work proceeds, they in fact arise out of an elaborate theoretical system that, in terms of the culture, is of relatively recent origin.

Nature, of course, has many other meanings than simply the objects of science, not all of which are strictly compatible. These usages often continue pre-modern conceptions of nature, translated into contemporary terms. In urban societies, for example, an important meaning of nature is that aspect of the social and economic unity that lies outside the metropolis, either conceptually or geographically—nature, in this context, is defined in relation to (or even in opposition to) the physical and social organisation of the city. In another usage, 'nature' refers to the realm of aesthetics—that is, to the world of sensory experience, valorised and structured according to contemporary criteria. Yet again, it may refer to the subjective world, the realm of private experience or of inner or spiritual life, also formed in relation to social and cultural influences. These ideas of nature may carry connotations of order, harmony and tranquillity, or they may suggest wildness and chaos. Whichever is the case, in all of them nature is situated firmly within culture. It is considered to possess both meaning and value, which themselves arise exogenously, from aesthetics, ethics, economics, religion and so on.

Nature, however, may be understood not just from within culture but as opposed to it. This quite different, much broader meaning is equally familiar but of greater importance for our present purposes. It is claimed by some that the distinction between nature and culture is a fundamental ontological fact[9], although, as we shall see, this view is by no means universally accepted. The conception of nature as standing in opposition to culture is important here because the existence of a radical distinction between the two is assumed by both of the sides in the animal experimentation debates. For the case of science, this is obvious: objectivism itself presupposes a radical disjunction between theoretical formulations and their objects. But the opponents of the scientists mark off the realm of nature from that of culture just as rigorously, albeit in a somewhat different manner: for them, animals have their own sphere of existence with its own integrity, autonomy and, possibly, values. For the scientists, the division is not a problem: it is a simple fact of existence. For the anti-vivisectionists, an abiding issue remains the possibility of a reconciliation.

In this latter sense, nature is not just an effect of culture. Quite the contrary, it is the conceptual representation of that which lies beyond culture and thus strictly outside the domain of language and communication. Here, nature is defined in relation not to politics, aesthetics or other constituents of culture but rather to culture as such. Thus, we refer to plants and animals, lakes and mountains, physical and organic and even psychological processes that we regard as independent of cultural processes as 'nature'. Despite the fact that this usage is employed frequently and easily in everyday life, it contains in fact quite a difficult, and apparently paradoxical, idea: nature in this sense is the obverse of culture, as it is conceived within it; it encompasses everything outside human society and therefore not strictly expressible in language. In perhaps more familiar terms, it is the 'environment' of culture and society.

The concept of the environment has, in recent years, entered the language of everyday discourse. While the term itself is relatively new, however, the idea underlying it is not. On the contrary, the problem in relation to which the concept was developed is truly a universal one. Every cultural configuration must arrive at some method for formulating the world that lies outside its boundaries, for thereby its own limits are established, along with the context within which its meanings are created.[10] At the level of epistemology, the problem has an apparent paradoxical character, for it involves the formulation of what by definition lies outside the domain of social expression—of articulating the ineffable, so to speak. Accordingly, in most cultural contexts, the problem is approached via other routes—through aesthetic and religious media, for example. In the age of science, however, this kind of solution is no longer tenable, especially in view of the implicit claim of scientific thought to be universal. Instead, the theoretical concept of environment was introduced to preserve the boundaries of culture without compromising the object domain of science.

The notion of the environment—first introduced in about the 1820s—was a haphazard but nonetheless largely workable solution. The environment comprised, in a loose sense, the surroundings of culture and the social world. It was defined in terms of, and hence existed only in relation to, them. Reflecting this, it was able to preserve the tension between that which could not be described precisely (because of its alien character) and the object of scientific investigation at its many points of intersection with human experience. The term was, and remains, useful in political discourse; as a rigorous theoretical concept, however, it was deficient from the beginning. This has not always been recognised, although the continuing debates about the status of reality in modern physics have repeatedly emphasised this fact.

In recent years, the notion of environment has partially given way to a more specific and in some ways more limited concept—that of 'ecology' or 'ecosystem'. The theoretical framework within which this concept arises is that of systems theory and cybernetics, which itself arose in the context of investigations into the structure of human communication. 'Ecology' is the study of the structure and function of dissipative, complex systems—which may include populations of plants or animals, or even human institutions—in relation to the environmental contexts within which they occur. With the help of the techniques of systems theory, ecology has become a major field of contemporary study.[11]

The weakness of the concept of ecology is that it fails to resolve the epistemological paradox implicit in the concept of nature from which it arises. Furthermore, it is required to operate at such a high level of generality that it sometimes sacrifices even qualitative detail. For example, it is designed specifically to encompass complex arrangements of very diverse elements that are assumed in advance to constitute a whole. However, often not only is the form of the interactions between specific variables imperfectly understood, but even the identities of the elements themselves may be questionable. In spite of this, it must be admitted that the theories that have been developed in relation to the concept of ecology are also often very suggestive and attractive. Their greatest attractiveness in fact lies, perhaps ironically, in the central position of the very concept with which they have most difficulty—that of totality itself, which is systematically excluded from the more conventional theories. In addition, their ability to mobilise diverse theoretical traditions, such as those of mathematics, engineering, communication theory and economics, have contributed to their popularity. But perhaps of greatest significance for the contemporary public debates is the stress that is placed in discussions of ecological systems on the notion of crisis.

The concept of 'crisis' was originally a medical one that became applied metaphorically to societies and to economies. In the language of ecology, a crisis is a process or state in which the integrity of an underlying structure is threatened. In the context of the debates about animal experimentation, the notion of an ecological crisis is an important one. For in spite of its apparent formulation as an epistemological concept, the idea invariably involves an attribution of values to the natural world. What is more, both the conviction that there exists an ecological crisis and the imperatives that are supposed to follow from it have achieved widespread agreement, if not absolute unanimity. The arguments themselves are, of course, very familiar: it is very widely understood that the combined impact of technology and industrial development have disturbed the equilibrium of various ecosystems comprising large populations of plants and animals; in some formulations the entire biosphere is at risk. In fact, so widely is this position held that even to question it is today widely regarded as politically and socially harmful.

On the face of it, the question of the existence of an ecological crisis would seem to be a purely factual matter that could readily be either verified or refuted by means of adequate data. This is not, however, the case. On the one hand, it is impossible to prove the existence of a state of crisis unless the structure and dynamics of the system in question and its conditions of stable operation can be specified in rigorous detail, and such knowledge is not yet available to us in relation to ecological systems. Without such knowledge, the hypothesis is reduced to an expression of an aesthetic or religious intuition or to a reflection of the inner conditions of the cultural formation itself. On the other hand, issues that have become matters of pressing and sometimes celebrated contemporary concern are not obviously new in an historical sense. Urban pollution was, if anything, worse in previous times; the rural environment was ravaged without restraint and many species were eliminated through hunting or specific agricultural practices. It is not obvious why people today should be especially concerned for the continued existence of sperm whales or snowy eagles or particular species of orchids when a hundred years ago their extinction would generally have gone unlamented. Further, it is a puzzling fact that concern for the integrity of the environment is highly variable in social terms, with those countries and the populations within them that are most affected often showing the least interest.

The concepts of environment and ecosystem are scientific in origin. However, the 'ecological crisis' is not primarily a matter of science: it is first of all a cultural crisis. It represents a formulation of questions and doubts that have developed regarding the whole project of the domination of nature, of which the Western economies as well as technology and—at least in its most familiar form— science are a part. To be sure, the technical details regarding the exhaustion of natural resources and, more recently, hypotheses about the 'greenhouse effect' and the destruction of the ozone layer are relevant and important. However, and this is the point, they could not on their own have created the perception of crisis or the committed concern for the long-term future of the environment. These responses are those of culture and society, and give expression to cultural concerns that are very deep-seated. They draw on a historical tradition, but the terms of their formulation are determined by the contemporary conditions of knowledge and discourse about the natural world.

The notions of ecology and environment have been given particular emphasis here because they form the most cogent and plausible contemporary formulation of the nature–culture distinction, a distinction that is central to the perspectives of both the scientists and their interlocutors. As mentioned, the fundamental status of the disjunction between nature and culture has been questioned recently, from several points of view.[12] In general, however, the critiques that are extant do not address in detail the question of science itself; indeed, in some formulations, science is treated with unconcealed contempt and the notion of objectivity is even declared obsolete. There are problems with the distinction and these have potentially significant implications for the practice of science; furthermore, they bear crucially on the place and role of animals. However, this does not invalidate the existing achievements of science and should not prevent its continuing development.

Animal Liberation

Let us return specifically to animals. From the point of view of the categories of culture, nature and environment where do animals stand?

There are several possibilities, which depend on the social and theoretical context within which the problem is formulated. Animals may in fact occupy a number of different locations. In tribal societies, for example, the species difference of non-human animals was recognised and respected. Animals were understood to inhabit their own domains, within which they possessed both inherent wisdom and a history; indeed, through totemic mechanisms, the specific knowledge of animals of their environments was adapted and applied to the organisation and classification of human societies. At the other extreme, in modern societies, animals are rarely recognised as possessing any special integrity of their own. For example, as food or as raw materials for other industries they are merely objects of utilitarian interest for humans in the conduct of their daily lives. As domestic pets, they fulfil limited cultural and psychological roles for their owners. In a large variety of other uses—horse racing, bull fighting, the employment of dogs for the assistance of the blind and so on—they are transformed into mere devices for securing human pleasure and comfort. Interestingly, game hunting—a less common form of relationship to animals, now actually banned in many countries because of its perceived 'inhumanity'—is one of the few instances in urban societies in which animals are regarded as possessing, by virtue of their species difference, a unique and autonomous sphere of existence that forms the basis of their interactions with humans.

What about the animals of science? Where are they located in the theories of both the scientists and the anti-vivisectionists? Here, the familiar formulations are somewhat misleading. From the point of view of science, animals are essentially no more than natural objects. They are, like atoms and molecules, the raw material for scientific research. To be sure, they may excite our curiosity and interest, but nonetheless they have no intrinsic value of their own: they exist primarily to serve human purposes. Accordingly, they belong on the side of environment. This, of course, it must immediately be said, does not prevent individuals from developing their own views about the value of animals. However, what is decisive for the practice of science is not the personal dispositions of individual scientists but the place that animals occupy systematically in the theory.

From the anti-vivisection perspective, things are very different. Non-human animals are regarded not merely as objective facts but as the subjects of values; indeed, at least at the outset of any discussion, before additional hypotheses have been introduced, their intrinsic value is assumed to be the same as that of humans. This means that their location is properly not in the environment but in culture. As a result, it is argued, they should be regarded as proper subjects of, and where appropriate, they should receive the protection of, the various cultural constructions of human society, such as systems of law and ethics.

It can be seen from our previous discussion that, in fact, neither point of view can provide an adequate account of the problem. Insofar as they are objects of science, animals already occupy a place in the culture—or, more precisely, in the theoretical system to which we refer, under the rubric of science, as 'nature'. Thus, nature itself cannot be adequately conceptualised as environment. Similarly, to the extent that they are considered to possess their own specific character and their own intrinsic value, animals must be regarded as separate from human culture. But if this is the case, their values must arise somehow exogenously: the only alternative is for animals to reside in a part of nature that intersects with culture—that is, in a region that, while still subject to the determinations of culture, remains radically separate from it. In other words, from both points of view, non-human animals must occupy both sides of the putative divide between culture and nature.

With this apparent paradox we can begin to see just how much is at stake in the animal liberation debate. What is at issue is not simply whether it is right or wrong—as concluded from an examination of either consequences or duty—to carry out scientific research on non-human animals. Rather, what is under discussion is the nature of nature itself—what it is, how it is known and what its relationship should be to both culture and environment.

Let us try to make the questions more precise. Animal liberation is not a theory of animals. It is not science. Indeed, it is not even concerned with knowledge. It is a radical attempt at initiating a reconsideration of the boundaries between nature and culture, between society and its 'environment'. The main protagonists do not, of course, express their project in this way, a fact that is in itself, as we shall see, highly significant—the insights and formulations of the animal activists have been limited by the system of discourse within which they have operated.

The concerns of science are very different from those of the anti-vivisectionists. Science seeks first of all to explore the theoretical system according to which it is postulated that the real world is structured. This system is linked to a semantics—a theory and a set of techniques for establishing the empirical relationships, and defining the experimental reality. In this system, animals are no more than biological phenomena: they are 'experimental systems' or examples of specific kinds of organisation. Accordingly, they may be 'sampled', 'studied' or maybe—in the rather curious, quasi-religious language that is adopted in a rare departure from the normally uncompromising hard-headedness of science—they are 'sacrificed'. For the anti-vivisectionists, by contrast, animals are cultural subjects of independent value; they are capable of sentience and suffering. They are not sampled or studied; they are 'killed', 'maimed' or even 'tortured'.

The scientists are interested in the pursuit of knowledge—as it is defined within their theoretical system. Their opponents, while they may value such knowledge, are concerned primarily—often implicitly and in an inchoate form—with a critique of the cultural forms that underpin the whole scientific enterprise.

Thus, the two approaches belong to quite different theoretical systems. In the one case, the subject matter—the domain of objects—has been constituted in the process of the development of an intricate theoretical system; in the other, it has emerged out of a tortuous process of cultural reflection on, and criticism of, science. Science and animal liberation, therefore, embody two different and contending theoretical systems, with different objects, different goals and different standards of validity and truth. In the language of the modern philosophy of science, the two theoretical frameworks constitute contending 'paradigms' or 'problematics'. It may not be going too far to suggest that they diverge so widely as to be truly 'incommensurable'.

The problem is an ethical one, in the broadest of senses. Put plainly, what is at issue is the conception of nature that we as a society should adopt. It is a discussion about the proper site of the boundary surface between nature and culture. It is a debate about our fundamental goals and values.

Under these circumstances, it is not surprising that communication between the two sides has been difficult. The scientists and the animal rights activists are talking about different things and in different ways. This is in spite of the use of a common philosophical language and the apparent dependence on arguments that are structurally very similar. In fact, the language of philosophical ethics has actually hindered understanding in this case rather than facilitating it. Before concluding, it is appropriate to return to the consideration of the ethical discourse itself to see how this has occurred.

Ethics and Communication

As we have seen, both sides formulate the arguments in support of their cases in the common language of philosophical ethics. This creates the impression that they are addressing similar problems. However, both the questions that are being asked and the theoretical agenda that is being followed differ in fundamental respects. The depth of this divergence, furthermore, is not generally appreciated—least of all by the protagonists themselves. Indeed, the public discussions about animal experimentation and the attempts on both sides to justify their positions have conspicuously failed to clarify the nature of the disagreement. The reason for this failure lies substantially in the nature of the bioethical discourse itself.

It is well-recognised that the theoretical starting point of an argument may determine, or at least limit, its final outcomes.

Accordingly, it is not difficult to appreciate that, in the case of ethical analysis, a given perspective may not have available to it all possible conclusions. More specifically, the functions of ethical debates should include, in principle, the clarification of values and the identification of assumptions underlying a particular hypothesis or proposed course of action. In cases where the ethical perspective that is applied incorporates presuppositions that bear on the actual subject matter of the analysis to be undertaken, it is likely that the realisation of these goals will be compromised. The debates about the ethics of animal experimentation provide an example of such a circumstance.

We have discussed some of the assumptions that are implicit in ethical theory. We have seen how the systems of ethical analysis that are associated with it were products of the same process of 'enlightenment' that gave rise to the scientific project of the domination of nature. Because they therefore share many of the presuppositions of science, where the validity of the assumptions underlying the latter are potentially in question, the ethical discourse too is thrown into doubt.

As discussed above, the theoretical project of the Enlightenment was directed by its underlying social goal: the liberation of mankind from his self-imposed immaturity (as Kant put it). As previously described, to realise this goal, both the achievements of science and, more importantly, its methods were to be applied universally for the development of society. For ethics, this meant that a system of thought was sought that could embrace all ethical values, or, at least, could provide a method for resolving ethical problems. In either case, through the judicious application of reason, a technique or set of techniques had to be available that could guide ethical choices. While the task was a difficult one in the execution, the underlying principle remained straightforward: the very definition of morality became identified with reason; virtue itself was, in the words of Toussaint, 'fidelity in fulfilling the obligations imposed by reason'.

The achievement of an apparatus with such a universal application naturally required its formulations to be constructed at a very high level of generality. This meant that the real human situations had to be abstracted and formalised, just as in science; that is, they had to be stripped of their temporal nuances and any unique features derived from personality or context. This led, again analogously to science, to an objectivistic conception of values—that is, to a conception of values the nature and existence of which were assumed to be independent of the constitutive processes of theory and subjectivity. As a result, the ethical discourse that emerged, and which continues to underlie contemporary bioethical thought, came to rely upon a particular conception of language as an instrumental device, a mere vehicle for the expression of ideas, external to ethics itself. In other words, language itself was presupposed and employed only as a means. This led, on the one hand, to an inability to recognise the ethical premises inherent in language and the linguistic interchange, and on the other to the neglect of the role of language as the theoretical medium of ethics in the formation of new values.

This account provides further insight into the deficiencies in the communication between the two sides in the animal experimentation debate. The situation is paradoxical. Both the scientists and the anti-vivisectionists adopt approaches to the analysis of the problem of animal experimentation that share fundamental assumptions about both knowledge and the objects of knowledge. At the same time, however, the thrusts of these analyses and their philosophical objectives are widely different—so different, in fact, that they must be considered to be addressing different problems. The inability of the two sides to communicate is a deep-seated problem. The obscurity of the debates is due to the fact that the fundamental divergence has been concealed by an equally fundamental common attitude to nature.

******

The basic issue at stake in the animal liberation debate is the way in which nature ought to be regarded and that this has been placed on the agenda for reasons that are themselves cultural in origin. I have tried to emphasise that traditional formulations that rely on the radical disjunction between nature and culture are no longer tenable—not because of a putative metaphysical innovation but because of the transcendental conditions of sociality and discourse.

This conclusion, it should be noted, does not preclude the continuing practice of science. The fact that we think through thought does not make objectivity impossible. Our knowledge may be true even if the object of that knowledge is both socially constituted and multifaceted in its structure. Nor does this commit us to an anthropocentric ethics, in which all that is non-human is valueless. On the contrary, clarity about the nature of our reflections ought to facilitate a deeper understanding of the ethical status of the natural world.

Nonetheless, these fundamental questions at this stage remain open. The debates that follow will need to address them, by means of methods of analysis that are not compromised in advance by commitments to the objects of their scrutiny. They will need to consider, for example, the epistemological status of living things; they will need to consider the ways in which the relationships between organisms and their environments are formed and represented in language; and they will need to consider the nature of science itself and the ethical consequences that follow from it.[13]

These are deep problems, which have often been shunned by practising scientists—not because the intellectual resources for addressing them are lacking but because they are simply considered to be too far from the mainstream of actual scientific work. The debates about animal experimentation have shown that such basic questions cannot be avoided, because they carry direct implications for the understanding of the natural world. But nor should they be, for their elucidation promises to supply us with even greater depth and richness of understanding.

Notes

1   RD Ryder, 'Speciesism in the Laboratory', in P Singer, ed., *In Defense of Animals* (New York, Harper & Row, 1986), pp. 77–88.
2   J Turner, *Reckoning with the Beast* (London, Johns Hopkins University Press, 1980); S Sperling, *Animal Liberators: Research and Morality* (University of California Press, 1988).
3   See, for example, MA Fox, *The Case for Animal Experimentation* (University of California Press, 1986).
4   See, for example, P Singer, *Animal Liberation* (New York Review, 1975); T Regan, *The Case for Animal Rights* (University of California Press, 1984); G Langley, ed., *Animal Experimentation: The Consensus Changes* (London, MacMillan, 1989).
5   J Habermas, *Knowledge and Human Interests* (London, Heinemann, 1972).
6   PA Komesaroff, *Objectivity, Science and Society* (London, Routledge and Kegan Paul, 1986).
7   cf. P Singer, *Animal Liberation*. But see also RD Ryder, *Animal Revolution: Changing Attitudes towards Speciesism* (Oxford, Blackwell, 1989).

8   A MacIntyre, *After Virtue* (London, Duckworth, 1982).
9   C Levi-Strauss, *Elementary Structures of Kinship*, ed. by R Needham and tr. by JH Bell, R Needham and JR von Sturmer (Boston, Beacon Press, 1969).
10 See N Luhmann, *Ecological Communication* (Cambridge, Polity, 1989).
11 See, for example, RE Ricklefs, *Ecology* (Middlesex, Nelson and Sons, 1980).
12 J Derrida, *Writing and Difference* (Chicago, University of Chicago Press, 1978); also S Griffin, *Woman and Nature: The Roaring Inside Her* (New York, Harper and Row, 1978).
13 There is already in existence a considerable literature from which the reconsideration of animal experimentation might proceed. See, for example, H Jonas, *The Imperative of Responsibility* (Chicago, University of Chicago Press, 1984); AN Whitehead, D Sherer and T Attig, eds, *Ethics and the Environment* (Edgeworth Cliffs, NJ, Prentice-Hall, 1983); EC Hargrove, *Foundations of Environmental Ethics* (Edgeworth Cliffs, NJ, Prentice-Hall, 1989).

CHAPTER 4
Sexuality and Ethics in the Medical Encounter

Two personal experiences illustrate some key issues concerning medicine and the body. One was at a Women's Health Day organised by a community health centre, at which I had been asked to give a talk about menopause and the experiences that women describe. At the conclusion of the talk, comments and questions were invited. A woman in the audience stood up and declared with undisguised intensity: 'No woman can know the pain a man experiences when he is kicked in the balls; no man can understand the pain a woman feels when she is going through menopause!' Then she sat down, to stunned, if somewhat embarrassed, silence.

The other incident occurred some years earlier. I was a junior hospital resident, exhausted from overwork and anxious to see my family. The last task for the day was to complete admission procedures for a middle-aged truck driver with an illness of uncertain cause producing progressive muscular weakness. The interview began routinely as I sought to record the history in a formal and logical manner. However, the patient responded to my questions only slowly and with imprecision. I became abrupt and aggressive. He became even less articulate, fumbling for words, unable to provide the most basic information. My body ached with tiredness and frustration, and I did not conceal my irritation. Then, in a moment of almost apocalyptic impact, I looked up from my page and for the first time directly met his gaze. What I saw disarmed and humiliated me. This man, burly, weather-beaten, his body marked by years of labour, no doubt once confident and assured in his own setting, was perched demurely on the edge of the hospital bed, feeble, emasculated, transfixed by fear and apprehension. His eyes divulged a softness and vulnerability that contrasted brutally with my own uncompromising harshness. In that instant, encountering him face to face, I recognised how little I knew of pain, uncertainty, terror. I glimpsed, in that moment, the depths of confusion and turmoil his illness had provoked, and I saw how wide of the mark my formal interrogation had been. It was a moment for me of insight, of transformation, of abruption, from which no escape was possible.

These two events, I believe, illustrate both the complexity and the perplexity inherent in discussions of sexuality and the clinic. The first, which was no doubt slightly overstated for the purposes of rhetoric, contains striking claims, some of which perhaps did not occur explicitly to the woman who made the statement. It raises questions about the gendering of experience and the possibility of empathy, about the nature—and indeed the possibility—of clinical medicine. The second shows how precariously balanced even apparently routine medical interactions can be. The bare, scientific discourse that constitutes the manifest content of much of medicine is often no more than a patina, a disguise or a vehicle, for other discourses—about the body, its history and its experiences. My shame and my tears showed me that the medical relationship can only be partially understood in terms of its technical functions: it is also, immanently, an ethical encounter involving embodied, suffering subjects.

In this chapter I wish to take up some of the themes raised in these examples and to explore some aspects of the role of sexuality in clinical medicine. I intend to argue in favour of three main claims. First, I shall argue that clinical medicine is concerned profoundly with bodies and their meanings. Bodies enter the clinic in various, sometimes contending, ways; indeed, there are many bodies—and discourses of the body—in the clinic. Accordingly, despite the official rhetoric, all medicine is, in a sense, concerned with sexuality. In arguing for this thesis, I shall adopt a rather broader notion of sexuality than is perhaps usual, which I shall explain in detail. Second,

I shall claim, once again in opposition to familiar viewpoints, that the doctor's body is not irrelevant to the therapeutic process, but rather plays a crucial and inescapable role within it. The doctor's body enters or inhabits the clinic in various ways, participates in communication and facilitates the therapeutic process. Here, my focus will be not on misuses of the clinical interaction but on its subtle, internal anatomy. Third, I shall argue that this interpretation of clinical medicine, as an intervention in a field marked by sexuality, raises fundamental issues of ethics and basic questions about the nature of medicine in general.

Sexuality in Clinical Medicine

In the official discourses of medicine, a rather narrow concept of sexuality is applied, restricted largely to sexual practices and identities.[1] An emphasis is placed on particular conceptions of 'healthy' sexuality, of putative pathological disruptions of it, and on therapeutic techniques to rectify such disruptions. Pathology is understood as arising out of relationship problems and hormonal or other biological factors. 'Treatments' are conceived as consisting of either pharmaceutical interventions—Viagra, testosterone, oestrogens[2]—or psychological techniques ('psycho-sexual counselling'). While there is good evidence that these remedies are sometimes efficacious in relation to the problems they are addressing, the framework in which sexuality is viewed—no matter how liberated it seems—remains partial and limited; as we shall argue, it captures only a very small part of what constitutes sexuality, and the role that it plays, in the clinic. In particular, it entails some fundamental omissions: it excludes from consideration, except in the most conventionalised, fragmented and attenuated sense, the body of the patient; it omits the fragile meanings written into the physical experience of illness and of the medical encounter itself; and it omits in its entirety the body of the doctor. In general, it omits the extraordinariness of medicine, which in a sense defines its specificity. This extraordinariness, commented on widely in the past, has been described well by Katherine Young at the beginning of her valuable book on the phenomenology of bodily experiences in medicine:

> Consider what transpires. I walk into a room, take off all my clothes, and permit a perfect stranger to inspect my naked

body ... How does this come about? Why isn't it a trespass, a violation, an assault, at least an impropriety? It goes against our customs, sets aside the practices of civilised life, flouts propriety. What transformation, what reconstitution, of my sense of my self and my body allows this unlikely intimacy, the physical examination?[3]

At least part of the problem described in this passage arises from the fact that both medical practice and sexuality can be viewed in various ways. Medicine can be regarded as a technical practice on a complex physiological apparatus, as a means for enforcing social control, or as a practice of liberation from physical and psychological constraints. Similarly, sexuality can be seen as a purely private affair, as an elaborate device for protecting the established structures of power, or as an intimate, shared property of a social relationship. I shall argue that there is, in fact, no privileged discourse of sexuality and medicine, and that each of these interpretations contain some validity, but that, despite this multiplicity of discourses, it is possible to identify enduring themes of sexuality that underlie all clinical encounters.

Theories of Sexuality

The intelligibility of the world is constructed corporeally. In his work *The Phenomenology of Perception*, Maurice Merleau-Ponty described in meticulous detail the processes according to which I apprehend the world through my body. While I apprehend the world corporeally, he argued, it is an inescapable fact that my body is also a part of this world, an object in it. As he puts it in his later work *Signs*, my body

> is a thing among things; it is caught in the fabric of the world, and its cohesion is that of a thing. But because it moves itself and sees, it holds things in a circle around itself. Things are an annex or prolongation of itself; they are incrusted into its flesh, they are part of its full definition. The world is made of the same stuff as the body.[4]

It follows from these arguments—as Merleau-Ponty shows— that although my body, as it were, inhabits its own subjectivity, it is not a phenomenon of myself alone, in isolation. It is imprinted from the start with traces of language, culture, experience—how my body is handled and the interpretation put on that handling. As he puts it, '[w]henever I try to understand myself the whole fabric of the perceptible world comes too, and with it come the others who are caught in it'.[5]

This social context of the body is irreducible. There is no way to section off the body from itself, or the embodied self from the world around it. The body is part of a broad context, as Richard Zaner, also utilising the phenomenological idiom, explained:

> Throughout the spectrum of bodily gestures ... there simply is no way to separate an inside. Embodiment, thus, is itself a gestural contexture within a still wider context: the world of concretely environing other live beings, other persons, social life, and that of 'nature' ... Corporeality includes the self, the body, and the world. I am fundamentally locused within and by my central body and my surrounding zonal sphere of immediate bodily action and spatiality.[6]

The role of the social in the constitution of the lived body has been put in even stronger terms by other writers. The very contours of the body are established through markings that seek to establish specific codes of cultural coherence.[7] Referring to the work of Mary Douglas, who showed that in tribal societies, what constitutes the limit of the body is never merely material, but that the surface of the skin is systematically signified by taboos and anticipated transgressions, Judith Butler has argued that indeed the boundaries of the body should be understood, in a sense, as the limits of the social, and more particularly, the socially hegemonic.[8] Accordingly, the 'body is not a "being" but a variable boundary, a surface whose permeability is politically regulated, a signifying practice within a cultural field of gender hierarchy ...'[9]

The experiences of illness draw particular attention to these boundaries. Pain, and disease in general, exert a power that reverberates throughout the phenomenological field, disrupting intentional linkages and transforming the bodily senses of spatiality and temporality.[10] Like the body itself, this process of transformation, which is guided and shaped through the face-to-face interactions of the clinic, is not a purely private affair: rather, it represents a complex intertwining of the private and the public. A person comes to a doctor with a problem, a concern, a physical symptom. Typically, this is experienced as a disruption both in the order of her physical existence and in the social world, the inter-human world, she inhabits.[11] In practice, of course, no distinction is made between the two realms. As Merleau-Ponty pointed out, a sick person does not mime with her body a drama played out in consciousness, or present a public version of a private inner state.[12] The body is not just a facet of existence, or an external accompaniment to it: it expresses total existence; it is the incarnation of a worldly presence that is loaded with immanent meaning.[13] In this sense, the body is the primary fact, in relation to which familiar categories, such as body and mind, sign and significance, autonomy and intersubjectivity, are constructed as abstract moments.[14]

It is commonly claimed that, as a result of its use of the discourses of science, medicine ignores the subjective experiences of the patient and reduces her body to an 'object'. I shall argue in detail below that this view is based on fundamental misconceptions about the nature and structure of the body. In particular, it assumes that the body can be separated from the self on the one hand, and from culture on the other. This, however, is impossible: the three are inseparable. Like science itself, the body is a cultural accomplishment, arising out of the phenomenological field of personal experience and incorporating within its structures the complex sedimentations of intersubjective life.[15]

Since Freud, sexuality has been understood as suffusing every aspect of our lives—as including not merely the genitally directed drive, or even polymorphous routes to pleasure, but all the trajectories around which meanings are created in relation to embodied being. Indeed, the idea of sexuality contains even more than this: it includes also the conditions of possibility for such meanings in general, and the ways in which networks of intersubjectivity are inscribed within bodies and common languages are developed that permit mutual intelligibility.

The modality of the body that allows us to constitute sense and meaning in the space between bodies—the space of 'alterity'—is what, I propose, we understand in the broadest sense as sexuality. Sexuality is not simply the state of being male or female. It is not some specific difference. It is—as Emmanuel Levinas has put it—'situated beside the logical division into genera and species'. The difference between the sexes 'is a formal structure ... that carves up reality ... and conditions the very possibility of reality as multiple, against the unity of being proclaimed by Parmenides'.[16] Neither is the difference between the sexes the duality of two complementary terms, for two such terms presuppose a pre-existing whole. To say that sexual duality presupposes a whole is to posit beforehand a moment of fusion—for example, a fusion of the kind that is referred to as 'love'. But in a sense this omits exactly what is important, for '(t)he pathos of love ... consists in an insurmountable duality of beings. It is a relationship with what always slips away ...' A direct, 'voluptuous' contact occurs between the lovers. 'The pathos of voluptuousness lies in the fact of being two.'[17]

Sexuality is a general presence in the world, which is both subjective and objective, private and social. This general presence, this intertwining, is a fundamental fact of human existence; in it is projected our manner of being towards the world, towards time and towards other people.[18] It can never be transcended, nor shown up by representations, either conscious or unconscious; nor can it be understood or interpreted at a purely cognitive level. It is an atmosphere in which we are immersed, albeit one that is ambiguous and problematic.[19]

It is perhaps worth noting at this point that the conception of sexuality sketched here diverges in substantial ways from the popular contemporary formulation identified with the work of Michel Foucault. According to our view, there is no body prior to its cultural inscription, no materiality prior to signification and form.[20] And unlike in Foucault's conception, the irreducible, historical ambiguity of subjectivity, as simultaneously an empirical fact and a source of knowledge and meaning, is not merely displaced into an effect of power or technology.[21] To be sure, Foucault's picture of medicine and doctors as functionaries of an oppressive regime is a compelling one. However, the conclusion that discourses derive from power and themselves possess hidden power, and that meaning and truth are no more than effects of systems of discourse and power[22], is not only too strong but also too pessimistic. It excludes any possibility of meaning creation in dialogical or communicative settings and would eliminate the subversive potential within social relationships to reflect critically on them.

Commenting on Foucault's essay 'Nietzsche, Genealogy, History', Judith Butler points out that while Foucault maintains that the task of genealogy is to expose a body totally imprinted by history, forces and impulses with multiple directionalities are precisely what history both destroys and preserves through the event of inscription. As a 'volume in perpetual disintegration', the body is always under siege, suffering destruction by the very terms of history; conversely, history is the creation of values and meanings by signifying practices that require the subjection of the body.[23] The body, she argues, cannot be seen as 'a ready surface awaiting signification, but as a set of boundaries individual and social, politically signified and maintained'. Similarly, sex should be seen not as an interior 'truth' of dispositions and identity, but as 'a performatively enacted signification … that can occasion the parodic proliferation and subversive play of gendered meanings'.[24]

With respect to medical discourse specifically, Foucault's work has undoubtedly opened up a potent critique of medicine's affirmative and normalising function. However, much of medicine is not normalising and affirmative, but, with respect to individual experiences, critical and subversive, and this dimension is formally suppressed in his theory. The implications with respect to sexuality in general are similar: while the conception of sexuality as a locus of power exposes an undeniable, underlying 'disciplinary' function, it also ignores the fluid and changing nature of sexual identities[25], and denies sexuality's creative and critical social role. In particular—of particular importance for the content of this book—it eliminates the possibility of any constructive place for sexuality in the process of making sense of illness or in clinical communication itself.

Sexuality, it may be argued, is not an effect of meaning: it is a site of meaning creation, or even a condition of possibility of meaning. It is a moment of corporeality that is capable of being intersubjectively shared. It is the component of the corporeal world that overlaps culture and makes communication possible. Conceived in this way, sexuality lies at the foundation of clinical medicine, for medicine deals precisely with the meanings of illness in relation to the body. The experiences that bring a patient to a doctor signify a disruption in a corporeal world that is both private and shared. They are accessible to the doctor in their fullness because of the nature, and through the medium, of sexuality. The suffering of another cannot be understood through processes that are purely cognitive: what is required is a perception that is sexual in character, in the sense that it aims directly from one body to another. To understand the experience of another, if that is my aim, it is not enough merely to theorise it; it must in some way be brought into existence for my own body. To achieve this, however, may not be at all straightforward, as the comment of the woman at the Women's Health Day quoted at the beginning of this chapter suggests. Indeed, a disarming moment, an unexpected disruption, may be required to subvert the established presuppositions of the interactions and to allow the embodied experience of the doctor to become visible: it is possible that the detail of the silk pyjamas may have performed precisely this function.

Medicine as Objectification or Subversion

Some of these points may be elucidated by discussion of an example. Marie, a successful businesswoman in her early fifties, began to experience panic attacks almost exactly at the same time as she started experiencing menopausal symptoms, such as hot flashes, night sweats and breast discomfort; indeed, often it was not clear to her which was which. She also noticed a degree of clumsiness not previously present, and she found herself bumping into things or even falling over from time to time. These symptoms were disturbing and perplexing to her, especially as she had formerly regarded herself as confident and outgoing and had never previously experienced a serious illness. The attacks and the other symptoms rapidly increased in severity and frequency to the point where she found it almost impossible to leave her home.

At first hostile and defensive in the clinic, as she described the development of her illness she gradually became more open and relaxed. She related how, in recent months she had come to experience her body as ugly and offensive, to the extent that she could no longer bear to look at herself in the mirror. Certain foods exacerbated her discomfort, making her feel bloated, fat and misshapen; this would lead to an overwhelming 'closed in' feeling, followed by a rising sense of panic. Sexual relations with her husband revolted her, and she considered separating from him. As she talked, many other issues in her life came into focus: a drug problem with one of her children, financial difficulties, the prospect of unemployment. She has a strong fear of breast cancer, since both her mother and sister had died of it at a similar age. She related secrets she had never previously confided to anyone: a teenage pregnancy and abortion, guilt about a refusal to see her dying father, unfulfilled aspirations to study and to become a writer or a painter.

At the beginning of each visit, Marie would enter confident and impeccably dressed. She would discuss her secrets and her fears and invariably become tearful and distressed. Then she would compose herself and vanish for a week, or a month, or several months. Occasionally she would telephone with new thoughts she had had, or new information. Again and again, she would demand reassurance that her meanings were understood, and that her pain was shared. At times she was comforted, at times challenged and confronted. Her language was sometimes angry, sometimes rambling, sometimes poignant. Unanticipated and painful associations often erupted in the midst of sober, carefully argued medical, psychological or philosophical discourses.

For Marie, the changed experiences of her body associated with menopause had fractured a fragile equilibrium, the existence of which she had not previously even been aware of. This equilibrium had enabled her for many years to secure order and stability in the fields of meaning with which she orientated herself. The corporeal disruptions had created a space for doubt and uncertainty, and, in the context of the clinical discourse, produced two sets of effects: on the one hand, a sense of uncertainty and threat; on the other, the possibility of access to new, previously inaccessible meanings. In some cases, she was able to render these perspicuous—for example, she concluded that her breast discomfort evoked the long latent fear of breast cancer—while in others, the underlying dynamic remained obscure.

In relation to the previous discussion, Marie's case illustrates two points. The first is the fundamental observation, so often overlooked in clinical medicine, that the body constitutes an axiological system within which epistemological, ethical and aesthetic meanings and values arise.[26] Illness involves a process not merely of a heightened awareness of bodily experience, but—at least potentially—a critical process of dissection and reintegration of this experience; an important moment of the clinical dynamic is to promote and foster this process of revision and critique. The second point is that the clinical process can be at once supportive and protective, and threatening and undermining. In relations of alterity, the other is a living, caring presence that can share one's suffering and so offers affirmation and reassurance. However, at the same time it manifests itself as irreducible and infinite, marginal, unable to be encompassed. Indeed, this moment of disruption, of challenge, of 'ethical resistance', as Levinas calls it[27], is precisely what allows the specificity of an individual's experience to be grasped. The institutions of totality, including law, science and ethics, can only judge the individual as a universal 'I', as the instantiation of a universal rule. The other as marginal—as the face-to-face interlocutor—does not fit as a particular instantiation of totality's universals. Totality always speaks in the third person, singularity in the first person: it always has a name.[28]

Medicine is a practice of the body, which stands alongside other practices of the body in a given society. In comparison with sport, dancing, aerobics and so on, it has some special features. For example, in the relationship with a doctor, many conventional rules of physical relationships are suspended: the bounds of privacy, respected even in intimate relations between lovers, are shifted, and a stranger is granted access to secret recesses of one's body and psychic life. Nonetheless, the rules that do govern the conduct of a doctor are very strict. Transgressions occur, although what is perhaps truly remarkable is that these are, comparatively speaking, rare.[29]

The patient maps her symptoms and bodily experiences against the various discourses of the body. The interventions of the doctor are those neither of a mere technician nor of a disembodied sounding board. Instead, he or she acts as an embodied subject who can understand and respond to the suffering of the patient within the order of the body itself. This means that the therapeutic process is multifaceted: it may encompass pharmacological and other physical therapies, language and communication, and, maybe, a contribution from the contact involved in the physical examination. In this aspect of his or her work at least, the doctor is not a technician. He or she is the symbolic agent of the patient.

It is commonly argued that medicine involves the application of a unified, monolithic discourse that has the effect of 'objectifying'— and thereby controlling—the body of the patient. Katherine Young puts the argument for a fundamental objectifying function of medicine strongly:

> In the realm of the ordinary, the body is the self, the site of my experiences, the fulcrum of my movements, the source of my perspectives. I experience myself as embodied. In the realm of medicine the body is rendered an object. It is inspected, palpated, poked into, cut open. From being a locus of self, the body is transformed into an object of scrutiny.[30]

According to this view, medicine fabricates a body of its own by inscribing the lived body in a discourse of objectivity.[31] The physician imposes a technocratic perspective that comes to dominate the voice of the lifeworld and leads to 'essential requirements for mutual dialogue and human interaction' being impaired and distorted.[32] Other writers, following Foucault, have taken an even more strident view, arguing that the medical relationship can be understood as no more than another institution of power. Evidence for this is adduced from analysis of the ways in which women are presented in textbooks of medicine[33], and from the experiences of women visiting gynaecologists. This point is expressed potently by Terri Kapsalis, who closely observed a number of gynaecological consultations. She describes the case of 'Gerry', who is subjected to a painful procedure to enlarge the vaginal introitus prior to marriage: despite her vigorous protestations, doctor, nurse and mother collaborate to chastise and subdue her. Kapsalis concludes: 'The pelvic exam is in effect the staging of sex and gender, particularly the staging of femininity and female sexuality ... The attempt to make Gerry into an uncomplaining and unresponding object is in effect an attempt to make her into a prop for the physician's performance'.[34]

If the medical relationship is understood in this way, as a process of regularisation and objectification, instances in which patients assert themselves in their particularity must be explained as strategies of opposition to the totalising discourse. Examples of such strategies include 'distortions' and 'contaminations' of the clinical process, such as lack of 'compliance' with the recommendations of doctors and nurses, and the introduction of personal stories to interrupt the flow of the medical discourse. Viewed in this way, stories are particularly interesting, because 'sealed off from the ... realm of medicine, as events of a different ontological status ... they can be used to reinsert into medicine an alternate reality in which the patient can reappear in his own person without disrupting the ontological conditions of the realm of medicine'.[35] This construction is certainly compelling. However, another interpretation is possible: that these distortions and contaminations are in fact themselves at the centre of authentic clinical discourse. Medicine is not a unified discursive system that is subject to corruption by extraneous elements. The 'official' discourses found in medical textbooks do not faithfully represent what transpires between doctors and patients. Rather, medicine contains an assemblage of discourses that interact in uncertain ways. The therapeutic relationship cannot be exhaustively described under the rubrics of power and social control, even if they cannot be excluded as contributing factors to it. A critical part of the clinical process is also to contribute to the clarification of the meanings of embodiment, by elucidating and mapping the multiplicity of coexisting discourses and voices.

In fact, as already suggested, objectification in general is not an exclusive property of medicine or science but represents an irreducible aspect of cultural and psychological life. Particular forms of objectification—such as those of the natural and human sciences—are themselves cultural accomplishments.[36] In the realm of medicine, the historical evolution of the characteristic extant species of objectivity has been clearly documented. This process included the invention of the distinction between public and private, its application to the body, and the subsequent reinscription of the latter as an object of representation, contrasted to a newly constructed, etherialised subject. From the beginning, this development was an ambiguous one, never brought to completion. The vicissitudes of the cultural constructions of the body have been demonstrated graphically by Mikhail Bakhtin, who documented in detail the transformations in the meanings and structures of the body at the end of medieval times. Whereas before its inception 'the flesh was the immediate, the unmediated, site of desire and penalty'[37], in the image of the individual body that emerged, 'sexual life, eating, drinking, and defecation [had] radically changed their meaning: they [had] been transferred to the private and psychological level where their connotation becomes narrow and specific, torn away from the direct relation to the life of society and to the cosmic whole'.[38] In grotesque realism, Bakhtin showed, the body

> is presented not in a private, egotistical form, severed from the other spheres of life, but as something universal, representing all the people. As such it is opposed to severance from the material and bodily roots of the world; it makes no pretence to renunciation of the earth, or independence of the earth and the body ... [T]his is not the body and its physiology in the modern sense of these words, because it is not individualised. The material bodily principle is contained not in the biological individual, not in the bourgeois ego, but in the people, a people who are continually growing and renewed.[39]

The grotesque body is grandiose and exaggerated, not separated from the world by clearly defined boundaries, but blended with it, with animals and objects; not finished or closed, but subject to constant transformation and change.[40] This conception of the body gradually gives way to 'a new bodily canon', from which the boundless imagery found in the grotesque culture of all that 'protrudes, bulges, sprouts or branches off' has been eliminated. The new view presented a completely contrary picture of the body, as 'entirely finished, completed, strictly limited ... which is shown from the outside as something individual'.[41] The meanings attached to parts of the body—buttocks, belly, nose, genital organs—are transformed, sometimes reversed. In particular, symbolic meanings are extirpated in favour of individual, expressive ones:

> In the modern image of the individual body, sexual life, eating, drinking, and defecation have radically changed their

meaning: they have been transferred to the private and psychological level where their connotation becomes narrow and specific, torn away from the direct relation to the life of society and to the cosmic whole. In this new connotation they can no longer carry on their former philosophical functions.[42]

The new discourse, however, could never be fully purified; the discordant moments could never be completely extirpated. As Francis Barker has argued, a tension has remained

> because of the tremulous existence of the modern body which is spoken there at the same time as it is silenced ... The carnality of the body has been dissolved and dissipated until it can be reconstituted in writing at a distance from itself ... [T]he body is supplementary. Neither wholly present nor wholly absent, the body is confined, ignored, exscribed from discourse, and yet remains at the edge of visibility, troubling the space from which it has been banished ...[43]

The tension arises, in part, because therapeutic discourse is not a purely 'scientific' discourse. It involves not just description and classification of events, but also the creation and elucidation of meaning. The words, the sentences, the stories of patients convey significations simultaneously at many different levels. This fact, of course, has long been recognised by psychoanalytic thinkers. As Freud observed, '[t]he word of the patient is at once situation and expression of situation'.[44] And in the words of de Waelhens:

> The discourse of the patient has many dimensions, many levels, which ... look for each other and anticipate each other ... Each word, each thing, in addition to its immediate and certain sense, 'reaches beyond itself toward a sense that it seeks' ... Behaviour has multiple meanings ... These secondary and tertiary significations etc. are no longer simply rational in the usual defined sense ... Psychoanalytic therapy tries to make the language which structures the

unconscious speak openly ... to promote 'the emergence of the symbolic world into the world of reality'.[45]

The same point applies to all clinical medicine, for which the specificity of the experience of every individual patient is irreducible. It is not just a matter of describing a biological process or of identifying hidden motives. It is also a matter of 'listening to a meaning which goes against another meaning and which manifests itself first as a non-sense. Indeed, this non-sense is not at all deprived of meaning. Simply, this meaning contradicts the lines of comprehension which, at first, seemed to impose themselves'.[46] In the clinic, we are faced with discourse, with meaning and with communication. The therapeutic process seeks to unveil new or concealed meanings, and, 'by reopening it to the plasticity and nourishment of a once more creative history ... restore the dynamic aspect of significance'.[47] Thereby, like John Berger's 'fortunate man', the doctor may come to occupy a role replete with meanings and symbols:

> He is their own representative. His records will never be offered to any higher judge. He keeps the records so that, from time to time, they can consult them themselves ... He represents them, becomes their objective (as opposed to subjective) memory, because he represents their lost possibility of understanding and relating to the outside world, and because he also represents some of what they know but cannot think.[48]

Touch and the Physical Examination

The doctor's role, however, is not just a symbolic one. On the contrary, his or her physical presence plays a critical role in the clinical interaction. The contact between doctor and patient is not mediated by words alone; physical touch is also an important conduit for meaning. As with verbal and other non-physical forms of communication, this latter aspect of the clinical process—touch, as it occurs in the physical examination—may assist in facilitating understanding, or sometimes in obstructing it. It may arouse intense issues, and focus or release specific anxieties. In view of its potent and irreducible role, it is perhaps surprising that clinical touch has been largely neglected in discussions about medicine.

As in the broader discussion about the discourses of medicine, it has often been argued that the physical examination is primarily a tool for depersonalisation and dehumanisation. As said previously, according to this view, there is a conflict between the voice of medicine and the voice of the lifeworld. As said previously, it is medicine that emerges the victor, suppressing and objectifying the experience of the patient and disarticulating his or her body.[49] And as said previously, while patients passively cede their bodies to the realm of medicine, they nonetheless engage in occasional acts of resistance in which the spell is briefly broken—for example, a moment of inattention, an interruption, or an attempt to insert a personal narrative.[50]

Once again, however, this elaborate construction is wide of the mark. Although an analytic intent is an important component of it, the physical examination cannot be comprehensively described in instrumental, or instrumentalising, terms. The most obvious reason for this is that the 'instrument' of the examination is primarily the body of the doctor itself—his or her hands, eyes and other senses. Accordingly, the practice of the examination is itself a practice of the body, but a practice of one body involving other bodies. The examination is a means for exploration, but it also opens up new possibilities for communication. It aims not merely to define volumes and densities, but also to explore, to understand, to communicate. The doctor's hands are not merely utilitarian tools: they are also a means for constructing meaning, 'at home on a body', familiar even with 'wounds which had not existed twenty minutes before'.[51] The clinical touch is not a purely instrumental device. As Levinas describes in another context, neither its role nor its function can be narrowly defined. It aims at neither person nor thing. It respects otherness, but also transcends it. Occupying the space between biological matter and the construction of meaning, it maintains a deliberate and systematic ambiguity.[52]

Clinical touch may often play an important therapeutic role. Indeed, it may be not too extreme to postulate, using the language of sexuality itself, that the doctor's touch may have the quality of a caress.[53] To employ Levinas' formulation once again, the caress is 'a mode of the subject's being, where the subject who is in contact with another goes beyond this contact. Contact as sensation is part of the world of light'. The caress, however—like the medical touch—is ambiguous and non-utilitarian.

> The caress transcends the sensible ... The caress consists upon seizing upon nothing, in soliciting what ceaselessly escapes its form towards a future never future enough, in soliciting what slips away as though it were not yet. It searches, it forages. It is not an intentionality of disclosure but of search: a movement unto the invisible.[54]

It is not the softness or warmth of the hand given in contact that the caress seeks. The seeking of the caress constitutes its essence by the fact that the caress does not know what it seeks. 'This "not knowing", this fundamental disorder, is the essential ... The caress is the anticipation of this pure future without content.'[55]

A peculiar and characteristic intimacy occurs in and through the medical relationship that is at once a condition of its possibility and the key to any therapeutic efficacy. Both the social aspects of the relationship and the subjectivities of the participants are constituted within the flux of the interaction. This is a feature shared with the erotic relationship. Furthermore, like the latter, the clinical interaction incorporates what Levinas calls (and to which we have already referred) 'voluptuousity', a kind of brute contact between bodies that bypasses conventionalised social relationships to be able to establish its own realm of meanings.[56] Like the latter, it is closed, 'supremely non-public'[57], excluding third parties. It cannot be adequately characterised in terms of 'grasping', 'possessing' or even 'knowing'. After all, possession, knowing, and grasping are synonyms of power: if this were all the medical relationship were, like the erotic relationship, it could not continue to exist. But there is nothing of all this, or the failure of all this, in either eros or medicine. If one could possess, grasp and know the other, it would not be the other.[58] It is only by showing in what way eros differs from possession and power that I can acknowledge a communication in eros. It is neither a struggle, nor a fusion, nor a knowledge. It is a relationship with alterity, 'with mystery, that is to say, with the future, with what ... is never there, with what cannot be there when everything is there'[59]—not with a being that is not there, but with the very dimension of alterity.

In spite of common features, however, the medical encounter is not a relationship between lovers, and it is important to emphasise that a sharp distinction must be maintained between the two. Indeed, it is appropriate to acknowledge that the possibility of an analogy between clinical relationships and erotic entanglements is a sensitive one for some people, for whom the comparison of a doctor's touch with that of a lover might be disquieting. Furthermore, erotic elements can contaminate the clinic, not merely in blatant transgressions but also in more subtle, though perhaps not less damaging, ways. While the distinction must be maintained, however, it remains remarkable that there is no ready language to describe the kind of intimacy established in clinical relationships, and that the only model of physical intimacy available is that of the erotic, of lovers.

Eros Versus Ethics

This brings us directly to the question of ethics in medical practice. In relating the case of Marie and drawing attention to various facets of both the patient's experience and the clinical encounter, I have sought to emphasise that illness cannot be understood adequately as a purely isolated, existential event in the life of a conscious being, as is suggested by some phenomenological accounts.[60] Rather, the lifeworld of personal experience is also always a social world. In addition to constituting the site of sensation and sensibility, it is the place where corporeal meanings are shaped, and where one not only recounts one's stories, which may be multifaceted and conflicting, to another person, but actively shapes and reshapes one's subjectivity. Illness and the clinical encounter, therefore, always have a dual character: in both, personal experience and social life are intertwined, not as pre-formed entities but as dynamic processes. Accordingly, the clinical encounter is a continuous, mutual process of forming and reforming values; it is immanently a site of moral action.

To speak in these terms, of the clinical relationship as a site of moral action, is not to suggest that it can be understood in terms of two isolated, 'autonomous' individuals confronting each other around a negotiable set of moral values. Indeed, the relationship is not a reciprocal one: the other 'is not only an alter ego: it is what I myself am not'.[61] I do not initially posit the other as freedom, from which alterity would then be deduced, for 'with freedom there can be no other relationship than that of submission or enslavement. In both cases one of the two freedoms is annihilated'.[62] I do not posit another existent in front of me, I posit alterity. The clinical relationship starts from the premise of alterity, the quintessential encounter with otherness; ethics is that 'putting into question of my spontaneity by the presence of the other'[63], which fixes the point of alterity. In other words, ethics is not an outcome or epiphenomenon of the clinic: it stands at its foundation, as both a presupposition and a condition of existence.

The ground of the clinical relationship, then, is the lifeworld contact between patient and carer. This relationship is not independent of social and cultural accomplishments; neither is it subject to goals and principles developed exogenously to it.[64] It does not subserve a particular category of the good, and it is not the site of the fulfilment of normative rules for action. It is, rather, the site where values are negotiated, or trajectories of value-related action are mapped out in the primordial contact between two individuals. The microethical relationship is not unstructured, however. It is critically dependent on the discursive forms established in relation to the larger-scale social formation. These structures, which could include a covert commitment to existing institutional arrangements and power structures, form the framework in relation to which the lifeworld contact is articulated.[65] This means that irruptions of contending discourses are frequently seen—not as contradictions or contaminations, but as valid parts of the process of exploring the lifeworld implications of those discourses.

For example, in a patient whose father died of a heart attack at an early age, the simple act of taking the blood pressure evoked a response of confusion and panic. Or, more potently, in a patient complaining of weakness, the routine test of muscular strength that was performed—which involves the clinician asking the patient to resist force applied to particular muscular groups—produced a puzzling lack of cooperation from a patient, a women in her sixties. Weeks later, she related how disturbed she had been by the test, which for her had evoked the physical abuse she had experienced in her marriage. She described how she had, with difficulty, suppressed her own violent response. 'Never do that to a woman!' she advised me, though not without some evident embarrassment.

Resistance

The clinical relationship is not always supportive and affirmative. It can also be subversive and challenging. The confrontation with serious illness can be an experience of growth and development; indeed, this is a general phenomenon of illness or, even more generally, of perturbations in bodily experience. The experience of pain, the disruption of the manifold of everyday bodily life, dramatically draws attention to the body itself as a thing that was taken for granted and can malfunction. Small events in bodily life, however, may play a similar function, and to a large extent make up the stuff of daily clinical practice. Often, the doctor's role is to enable and facilitate understanding, to assist with the taming of bodily experiences, and with mapping and remapping the discourses in which the body is inscribed. He or she does this by standing as another embodied subject, brought into a relationship that is capable of suspending social assumptions, and of establishing direct contact that can develop innovative forms of communicative action.

Through the experience of illness, the structures of otherness and the boundaries of sense are put into question. The clinical process, including its therapeutic interventions, awakens new modes of embodiment and raises the possibility of new—often unsettling—meanings. Examples of this phenomenon occur daily in clinical practice. Two cases involving treatment with the androgenic hormone testosterone illustrate this point. The first concerns a man who commenced testosterone therapy for management of diminished sexual desire that was threatening his marriage. While a revival of sexual thoughts and interest did occur, to his consternation these were associated with a profoundly threatening sense of alienation from his own bodily sensations. For the first time in many years he felt able to express his emotions openly; however, this expression was at best only barely containable and on several occasions manifested itself as violent outbursts that took all, including and especially himself, by surprise. The second concerns a woman who undertook a similar treatment for the same reason. Although it is common for women to whom testosterone is administered for the purpose of improving vigour and sexual desire after menopause to report increases in both sexual interest and responses, it is well documented that many after a time decide to discontinue therapy. In this case, the patient explained her decision to discontinue treatment with testosterone on the basis that the sexual feelings she experienced with the drug were more genitally focused than she had known previously, causing her both surprise and bewilderment. She declined further treatment, saying that she did 'not want to experience lust like a man'. For both these patients, the treatment opened up the possibility of new modes of experience and new meanings, which were at once not only interesting and engaging but also puzzling and challenging.

The confrontation between the partners in the clinical encounter can be perplexing, threatening or productive; it can provide support and affirmation, or subvert and confront. Its function is not just the integration of experience, but also disintegration, questioning, anatomising. The moral exigency to which alterity gives rise is inherently unsatisfiable, because the other (that is, the doctor) cannot be thematised, objectified or totally defined. The face refuses to be contained; it remains infinitely transcendent, infinitely foreign.[66] This is the obverse side of the ethical relationship that subtends discourse: it is threatening, challenging, 'it puts the I in question'.[67]

Politics of Sexuality and Sexual Difference

We have been arguing that an analysis of the role of sexuality in clinical medicine reveals profound inadequacies in the dominant paradigms by which sexuality is understood. In particular, biological reductionist frameworks, conceptions focusing on sexual practices or identity, and formulations that regard sexuality as no more than an epiphenomenon of the social institutions of power, all fail to capture the rich and diverse nature of sexuality in medicine. Instead, we have suggested that discussions of sexuality should emphasise the ethical and intersubjective foundations of the clinical encounter and the multiplicity of forms of alterity it encompasses. The clinic is a site of critical interrogation of sexuality, understood in this broader sense as the intersubjective moment of corporeality. This interrogation takes place as a dialogue between two embodied subjects—not, however, as subjects constituted in isolation from each other and subsequently brought into formal communication, but as poles in a flux of alterity that differentiates into subjects in the dynamic of the interaction itself. The clinic encompasses many discourses that may contribute to this process.

It must be acknowledged, however, that like the other formulations of sexuality, this one too may have its limitations. For example, to regard gendered bodies not primarily in terms of sexual practices or identities but as representing different corporeal styles, as so many 'styles of the flesh'[68], may obscure important features of sexuality. In particular, it may understate the foundational role of sexual difference in cultural production, or the political implications of male or female identity.

It has been argued—for example, by the French philosopher and psychoanalyst Luce Irigaray—that in Western philosophy and culture, the feminine is conventionally apprehended as the underside or reverse of man's 'aspiration towards the light', as its negative, from the point of view of man, through a strategy dictated by masculine pleasure.[69] For her, women constitute a paradox within the discourse of identity itself: they are the 'sex' that is not 'one'. Within a masculinist, 'phallogocentric' language resting on univocal signification, they appear as a linguistic absence, a moment of unrepresentability. In place of the masculine categories of 'subject' and 'other' generated by the totalising signifying economy of phallogocentrism, the female sex occupies the place of the unconstrainable and the undesignatable.[70]

According to this radical view, the structures of knowledge—indeed, the conception of knowing itself—are contaminated from the beginning with the effects of sexual difference. If this is true, it may be the case that the discourses of the clinic—as various and complex as they are—are also already gendered, already compromised by the marks of phallogocentrism. The patient who declared 'Never do that to a woman' may have been responding to a sense that, at least in part, medical discourse demonstrates an ontological commitment that is tied, not trivially to a particular scientific or objectifying discourse, but to the whole structure and discourse of discourses. Similarly, the woman for whom the administration of testosterone evoked the experience of sexuality 'like a man' may have been reflecting on the formulation of sexual interest and pleasure as a problem or issue within a theoretical framework that defines in advance the terms of its own solutions.

The former point concerns the undeniable political aspect of sex and sexuality. For Foucault, the body gains meaning within discourse only in the context of power relations, and sexuality is a historically specific organisation of power, discourse, bodies and affectivity.[71] It is true that in a conception of sexuality that focuses not on identity but on corporeal styles and their meanings, neither knowledge nor power assumes pre-eminent significance. An emphasis on the direct transfer of meaning between bodies, on voluptuousity, shifts the focus from power and the products of sexual difference to the relation with the other to its own absence, and to the alterity of a sexually non-marked wholly other.[72] This view disputes the assumption that the body is indelibly marked with, and ineradicably formed by, a particular species of sexual difference, and that there is no possibility of recourse to a person, a sex or a sexuality that escapes the matrix of power and discursive relations that produce and regulate the intelligibility of those concepts for us.[73]

In supporting a view that we believe is consistent with the one expressed here, Judith Butler has argued that the substantive grammar of sex imposes an artificial binary relation between the sexes, as well as an artificial internal coherence within each term of that binary, and suppresses the subversive multiplicity of a sexuality that disrupts conventional heterosexual, reproductive and medico-juridical hegemonies.[74] According to Butler, the privileging of sexual difference itself conveys adverse political consequences—by identifying women with sex, the category of woman is conflated with the ostensibly sexualised features of their bodies, and this is used as an excuse to deny to women the freedom and autonomy supposedly enjoyed by men.[75] Following Nietzsche's claim in *On the Genealogy of Morals* that 'there is no being behind doing, effecting, becoming; "the doer" is merely a fiction added to the deed—the deed is everything', Butler goes on to propose a corollary 'that Nietzsche himself would not have anticipated or condoned': that '[t]here is no gender identity behind the expressions of gender; that identity is performatively constituted by the very "expressions" that are said to be its results'.[76]

Many Discourses, Many Bodies

Reality is not homogeneous and indivisible: it is complex and heterogeneous, internally divided, a mixture of otherness and sameness.

Truth is not a matter of a revelation of an essence, an interrogation of sameness: it is a dynamic process directed towards the apprehension of difference, the attempt to grasp what is other. The subject is not a unified entity, isolated and solitary: it is radically pluralistic, generated out of the experience of otherness or, more precisely, the alterity between self and other. The self, moreover—as we have argued—is not a thing: it is a relation, a relation to other embodied selves, to other modes of alterity, to the world. Our sense of exteriority, and of these relationships, is irreducible. The body—indeed, the myriad bodies 'that constitute the domain of gendered subjects'[77]—is not a ready surface awaiting signification: it is a product of a process of cultural construction, a signifier inscribed and rendered meaningful through the operation of contesting signifying practices.

We have discussed how the body of Western science and medicine is a historical accomplishment, the product of a complex cultural process itself marked by interruptions and contradictions. In the account offered by Bakhtin of the formation of the post-medieval body, the critical moment offered by the carnival gives way to linguistic differentiation, to 'heteroglossia', which becomes a feature of the emerging culture.[78] Indeed, today at least, heterogeneity, transformation and resistance are constant features of the body and bodily experiences. There is always a tendency for boundaries to be transgressed, and for the contents of discourses to be switched. What Bakhtin described in relation to the Rabelaisian body applies equally to contemporary times: '[a]ll that is sacred or exalted is rethought on the level of the material lower bodily stratum or else combined and mixed with its images'. This movement is 'directed into the depths of the earth, the depths of the body, in which "the treasures and most wonderful things lie hidden"'.[79]

Similarly, the jumbled voices Marie and other patients articulate in their discussions of illness are not indications of pathology: they are authentic presentations of their selves. The self today is concrete and pluralistic. All individuals occupy many roles—in work, in the community, in families, in intimate relations; all of us experience sadness and happiness, pleasure and pain. The unfamiliar experiences of the body in illness, menopause, puberty and ageing may—often with the guidance of clinical discourse—throw stable, predictable worlds into question, shatter their unity, and at once produce both an impression of chaos and confusion and the possibility of new meanings and values. The body, like the clinical discourse itself, is heterogeneous and fluid.

I have argued in this chapter that medicine is concerned immanently with issues of sexuality; that is, with the shared meanings that arise in relation to corporeal existence. Doctors and patients encounter each other as embodied subjects, and therefore within an ethical relationship. In the complex ethical topography of the clinic, all the ambiguities and perplexities of the broader field of sexuality are well represented.

The clinical encounter inhabits a space that is at once personal and social and that spans the sexual field in which both patient and doctor are immersed. It is diverse and differentiated; it must accommodate different roles and therapeutic strategies, and the different stories the patient may tell. Its unifying theme is the ethical presupposition on which it is built, the primordial responsibility that underlies all relationships. Both the concept of sexuality and that of ethics developed here oppose the notion of a single, totalising discourse based on presuppositions or principles exogenous to the interactions to which they refer, and they reject universal and universalising concepts of the body, of sexuality, of the good and of clinical discourse itself. Indeed, I have argued, it is one of the major tasks of the clinic to preserve a space within which critical reflection on the conventional structures of the body can be protected and promoted. This may seem like a wild aspiration in a time of intensifying technological hubris and political reaction, but in reality it represents no more than a reaffirmation of the traditional role of the clinic.

I opened this chapter by referring to two examples. One—from the Women's Health Day—was about the multiple alterities of the clinic, with an emphasis on the question of sexual difference. The other—the account of my personal experience while admitting a patient with progressive weakness—showed how, under the searing force of the face-to-face encounter, the technical discourses of medicine may be overwhelmed by the direct apprehension of the corporeal world of another. Together, these examples emphasise the diversity and fecundity of the questions raised within medicine by and about sexuality. It may also be seen that one of the primary tasks of the multiple discourses of the clinic is not to answer these questions, but to preserve and foster this diversity and fecundity.

Notes

1. See J Wiltshire, P Rothfield and PA Komesaroff, 'Introduction', in PA Komesaroff, P Rothfield and J Wiltshire, eds, *Sexuality and Medicine* (Xlibris, 2004).
2. For example, BR Komisaruk, C Beyer-Flores and B Whipple, *The Science of Orgasm* (Baltimore, Johns Hopkins University Press, 2006); RE Nappi, 'New Attitudes to Sexuality in the Menopause: Clinical Evaluation and Diagnosis', *Climacteric*, 10, Suppl. 2, Oct 2007: 105–8; S Kingsberg, 'Testosterone Treatment for Hypoactive Sexual Desire Disorder in Postmenopausal Women', *J Sex Med*, 4, Suppl. 3, Mar 2007: 227–34; M Redelman, 'A General Look at Female Orgasm and Anorgasmia', *Sex Health*, 3(3), Sep 2006: 143–53.
3. K Young, *Presence in the Flesh. The Body in Medicine* (Cambridge, MA, Harvard University Press, 1997), p. 1.
4. M Merleau-Ponty, *Signs* (Evanston, North-western University Press, 1964), p. 163.
5. ibid., p. 15.
6. R Zaner, *The Context of Self: A Phenomenological Inquiry Using Medicine as a Clue* (Athens, Ohio, Ohio University Press, 1981), p. 66.
7. J Butler, *Gender Trouble. Feminism and the Subversion of Identity* (New York, Routledge, 1990), p. 131.
8. ibid., p. 131.
9. ibid., p. 139.
10. D Leder, *The Absent Body* (Chicago, University of Chicago Press, 1990), pp. 80–1.
11. M Merleau-Ponty, *The Phenomenology of Perception* (London, Routledge, 1962), p. 159.
12. ibid., p. 161.
13. ibid., p. 165.
14. ibid., p. 166.
15. cf. M Polanyi, *Personal Knowledge* (London, Routledge and Kegan Paul, 1962); PA Komesaroff, *Objectivity, Science and Society* (London, Routledge, 1986).
16. E Levinas, 'Time and the Other,' in S Hand, ed., *The Levinas Reader* (Oxford, Basil Blackwell, 1989), p. 48.
17. ibid., p. 49.
18. Merleau-Ponty, *Phenomenology of Perception*, p. 158.
19. ibid., p. 168.
20. J Butler, *Gender Trouble*, p. 130.
21. J Habermas, *The Philosophical Discourse of Modernity* (Cambridge, MA, MIT Press, 1987), p. 270.
22. ibid., p. 276.
23. J Butler, *Gender Trouble*, pp. 129–30.

24 ibid., p. 33.
25 cf. J Rose, *Sexuality in the Field of Vision* (Verso, 1986), pp. 90–1.
26 See Chapter 6.
27 E Levinas, *Collected Philosophical Essays* (Dordrecht, Martinus Nijhoff, 1987), pp. 56.
28 ibid., pp. 194ff.
29 When they do occur, it must be recognised that they may cause profound damage. See Peter Rutter, *Sex in the Forbidden Zone* (Los Angeles, Jeremy P Tarcher Inc., 1986).
30 K Young, *Presence in the Flesh*, p. 1.
31 ibid., p. 5.
32 ibid., pp. 37–8.
33 T Kapsalis, *Public Privates: Performing Gynecology from Both Ends of the Speculum* (Durham, Duke University Press, 1997), p. 94 etc.
34 ibid., p. 14.
35 K Young, *Presence in the Flesh*, p. 42.
36 See PA Komesaroff, *Objectivity, Science and Society*.
37 F Barker, *The Tremulous Private Body* (Methuen, London, 1984), p. 63.
38 P Morris, *The Bakhtin Reader* (London, Edward Arnold, 1994), p. 236.
39 M Bakhtin, *Rabelais and His World* (Bloomington, Indiana University Press, 1984), p. 19.
40 ibid., pp. 26–7.
41 ibid., p. 320.
42 ibid., p. 321.
43 F. Barker, *The Tremulous Private Body*, pp. 62–3.
44 S Freud, *The Complete Psychological Works*, vol. X, tr. L Strachey (London, The Hogarth Press, 1974), p. 167.
45 A de Waelhens, *Schizophrenia. A Philosophical Reflection on Lacan's Structuralist Interpretation*, tr. W Ver Eecke (Pittsburgh, Duquesne University Press, 1978), p. 202.
46 ibid., p. 204.
47 ibid., pp. 197–200.
48 J Berger and J Mohr, *A Fortunate Man* (New York, Pantheon Books, 1976), p. 109.
49 K Young, *Presence in the Flesh*, pp. 32–3.
50 ibid., p. 33.
51 J Berger and J Mohr, *A Fortunate Man*, p. 18.
52 E Levinas, *Totality and Infinity* (Pittsburgh, PA, Duquesne University Press, 1969), pp. 258, 259.
53 L Irigaray, *An Ethics of Sexual Difference* (New York, Cornell University Press, 1993), pp. 185ff.
54 E Levinas, *Totality and Infinity*, p. 258.
55 E Levinas, 'Time and the Other', p. 51.
56 E Levinas, *Totality and Infinity*, p. 266.
57 ibid., pp. 263–4.
58 E Levinas, 'Time and the Other', p. 51.
59 ibid., p. 50.

60 See Drew Leder, *The Absent Body*; SK Toombs, *The Meaning of Illness: A Phenomenological Account of the Different Perspectives of Physician and Patient* (Boston, Kluwer Academic Publishers, 1993).
61 E Levinas, 'Time and the Other', p. 48.
62 ibid., p. 50.
63 E Levinas, *Totality and Infinity*, p. 43.
64 See PA Komesaroff, P Rothfield and J Daly, *Reinterpreting Menopause* (New York, Routledge, 1997).
65 See Chapter 2.
66 E Levinas, *Totality and Infinity*, p. 194.
67 ibid., p. 195.
68 J Butler, *Gender Trouble*, p. 139.
69 L Irigaray, 'Questions to Emmanuel Levinas: On the Divinity of Love', in R Bernasconi and S Critchley, *Re-reading Levinas* (Bloomington, Indiana University Press, 1991), p. 109.
70 J Butler, *Gender Trouble*, p. 9.
71 cf. ibid., p. 92.
72 J Derrida, 'At This Very Moment in This Work Here I Am', in R Bernasconi and S Critchley, *Re-reading Levinas*, p. 40.
73 J Butler, *Gender Trouble*, p. 32.
74 ibid., p. 19.
75 ibid.
76 ibid., p. 25.
77 ibid., p. 8.
78 M Bakhtin, *The Dialogical Imagination: Four Essays* (Austin, Texas University Press, 1992), pp. 259–75.
79 M Bakhtin, *Rabelais and His World*, pp. 370–1.

CHAPTER 5
The Medicalisation of Everyday Life and the Moral Space of the Menopausal Woman

Amelia, a 47-year-old lecturer in women's studies, has experienced a variety of symptoms she attributes to menopause—including hot flushes, headaches, tiredness and irritability—for more than a year. Despite her open mistrust of Western medicine and her conviction that hormonal therapy is primarily a device to promote patriarchal power and drug company profits, she now attends a menopause clinic and takes oestrogen therapy. Although this is successful in controlling her symptoms, her assessment of medicine and hormonal therapy is unchanged.

Brenda is fifty-nine and also suffers from menopausal symptoms. About five years ago, she attended an open day organised by a local menopause clinic to promote hormonal treatments. She listened to women who described how they had been rejuvenated by 'HRT' and subsequently commenced the treatment. Although it provided little relief, she persevered because of alleged beneficial effects for her bones and heart. Last month she was diagnosed as suffering from breast cancer and she has been told that a link between the treatment and the diagnosis cannot be ruled out. She blames the doctor for her cancer and is angry and resentful.

No matter what form it takes, medicine is regarded with ambivalence and suspicion, as are the doctors who practise it. This is hardly surprising: on the one hand, medicine promises relief from pain and disease and the restoration of health and vigour. On the other, the death rates for many diseases, like HIV and cancer, remain unchanged and there seems to be an endless series of reports about the harmful effects of drugs and other medical treatments. On the one hand, the doctor is entrusted with confidences and confessions of a most intimate kind; on the other, the relationship itself is formal and impersonal, with an explicit commercial content. On the one hand, the doctor is appealed to as an ally against the crushing weight of everyday life and the rigours of work; on the other, he or she is clearly a representative of privilege and power and a functionary of an elaborate and ruthlessly efficient system of social control.

Medicine lies on an invisible boundary between the private and the public, between personal freedom and social control, between the intractable demands of nature and the historically conditioned effects of culture. In recent years, the internal tensions within medical practice have been exposed in a series of potent critiques. Feminists, gay activists, philosophers and cultural theorists have subjected its philosophical and cultural presuppositions and its social origins and outcomes to relentless scrutiny. In particular, the disciplinary functions of medicine have been carefully analysed, including both the ways in which it helps to service the productive apparatus of society directly and the more subtle, indirect means by which it reinforces the complex ideological structures that regulate individual bodies.[1]

One of the most fruitful outcomes of this process of critical reflection has been the re-examination of the tendency of medicine and its institutions to view everyday life experiences through the lens of its own instrumental concepts. Birth and death, childhood and ageing, puberty and menopause, sexuality and body shape have all come to be regarded as physical states that can be described in scientific terms, classified in relation to health and disease and subject to technical intervention and manipulation. For example, menopause, a natural life event, has been reclassified by modern medicine as a disease state characterised by hormonal deficiencies and physical decay requiring pharmaceutical and other therapies to restore a healthy equilibrium.[2] The critical reassessment of medicine and bioethics has led to the reassessment and reinterpretation of menopause, and, conversely, the cultural ferment around the understanding of menopause has become an important site for innovative reflections on medicine. The analysis of the promotion and effects of hormonal therapies, of the operation, under the guise of mere 'technical' decision-making, of the institutions of medical and economic power, of the reduction of complex realms of experience and meaning into biological facts or their consequences—all of these reveal as much about medicine as they do about menopause. What is more, they reveal not just the limitations of medicine, but also its richness, diversity and subtlety.

Taking menopause as an example, this chapter seeks to examine the vicissitudes of clinical communication around everyday physical experiences. It explores the anatomy of the communicative structure of medical practice and the role of values in shaping the face-to-face interactions within the clinic. It examines the moral disorientation that sometimes occurs in relation not just to serious illness but to 'natural' processes of bodily transformation.

The Multiple Discourses of Medicine and Menopause

Carli is forty-three and scared of dying. She is unemployed. She can't sleep. All her life she has had to battle against prejudice directed at her racial background. She has never had children and doesn't know if she should regret that. She is tired; she is putting on weight; her marriage is under threat. When she comes to the doctor she says that she cannot understand what is happening to her: her body is out of control. She has tried herbal medicines, but they didn't work. She says that she felt she 'needed to nurture [her]self', so she took leave without pay from work—she never went back—and practiced meditation, yoga and aroma therapy. That hasn't worked either. She wants 'a measure of something', 'a way of organising and controlling' her experiences.

As discussed in previous chapters, contrary to the impression sometimes created by its critics, clinical medicine does not consist of a single unitary discourse. Rather, it is a complex of contending discourses. There are the discourses of science, anatomy and physiology, and of the pathological theories developed out of them; there are psychological, social and ethical discourses; and there are those of practical action—technical and moral—and of therapeutic interventions of various kinds. There is not one 'medical gaze', but many.

The same can be said of domains of ordinary bodily experiences, including menopause. There is no single discourse of menopause. Indeed, the concept 'menopause' is itself a complex one, referring to a multiplicity of theoretical and cultural perspectives on a variety of issues, from the biology of ageing to the philosophical understanding of death. Discussions of menopause may refer to biology or politics, hormones or feminism, psychoanalysis or social control, and when it comes to individual experiences, women provide widely varying accounts.

The contending themes of medicine intersect with those of menopause in unpredictable ways. In a particular case, the locus of these intersections is subject to the social and psychological context and to the value systems of patient and doctor. Values are of particular importance, despite the emphasis in medicine on technical, instrumental action. Indeed, interactions between doctors and patients are critically dependent on personal commitment and communication regarding issues of value: the two come together in a moral universe, or, as I shall term it, 'moral space', a conception that will be developed in detail presently.

As previously discussed, the (post)modern world is infinitely various and diverse. In place of fixed, unchallengeable criteria for judgement, there are contending perspectives. This world is—at least potentially—a place of unconditional freedom in which one may even acquire the ability to choose the nature of one's own subjectivity. Even the identity of the postmodern person is contingent and context dependent.[3] This is the world that Nietzsche was describing when he referred to the 'lack of order, arrangement, form, beauty, wisdom, and whatever other names there are for our aesthetic anthropomorphisms'. It is a world that is free of ethical or aesthetic presuppositions. In Nietzsche's words again:

> [H]ow could we reproach or praise the universe? Let us beware of attributing to it heartlessness and unreason or their opposites: it is neither perfect not beautiful, nor

noble, nor does it wish to become any of these things ... None of our aesthetic and moral judgements apply to it.[4]

Carli's discourse contains a miscellany of epistemological styles and questions of moral significance. The world of things and values she inhabits is under threat. Basic questions she has asked, or has avoided asking, throughout her life, thrust themselves forward at this time. Her moral space—the region within which she has made her decisions about relationships, work and children, and has interpreted her bodily experiences—is fragmented and disordered. The framework within which she once orientated herself with respect both to morality and truth now appears to her gratuitous and unworkable. In this setting, she seeks the assistance of the doctor. In the medical encounter she exposes herself—the questions, the doubts, the confusions about issues of value—and attempts to come to terms with her predicament.

Although the provision of such assistance is an ancient component of clinical practice, it is almost completely absent from contemporary accounts of the ethical dimensions of medicine. Indeed, despite their popularity and inherent interest, these accounts omit from consideration a large part of the many issues of values that preoccupy individuals in their daily interactions. The precise nature of these issues varies according to the setting. In the context of menopause, these issues include a wide range of questions concerning sexuality, ageing, death and the body, the relationship between the individual and society, the social functions of medicine and the roles of hormonal therapy as possible instances of patriarchal power. Both medical practice and the varieties of menopausal experience, therefore, are complex and multifaceted. To develop further the understanding of both of them, and of their interaction, it is necessary to pass to a closer examination of the moral dimensions of the clinical interaction.

Moral Space, Identity and Ethics

About a year and a half ago, Diedre, a 34-year-old landscape gardener with two young children, developed severe pelvic pain. Her gynaecologist assured her that nothing was wrong, but the pain continued and eventually became much worse, necessitating an emergency operation. There, it was found that she had benign tumours on both ovaries, and a ruptured cyst had led to the widespread dissemination of tumour material throughout the pelvis and abdomen. Another operation was required, which entailed the removal of both ovaries, the uterus and other tissue in the pelvis and abdominal cavity. After the operation, Diedre was devastated. She had no energy and was unable to work. She experienced intermittent pelvic pain, which always suggested to her the possibility of tumour recurrence. She attempted to contact the gynaecologist but was told repeatedly by his secretary that he did not need to see her again. Eighteen months later, Diedre seeks another medical opinion. She still has not returned to work and, indeed, remains largely confined to bed. Her life is limited, isolated and lonely.

People come to doctors for many different reasons. They may say that they merely seek information and advice about technical questions, for example. Often, as they talk, however, it becomes obvious that there is much more to it than this. The experience of the illness and the operation have shattered Diedre's world. They have destroyed her confidence in her body and in her relationships with others. She has lost her job, her marriage, the overall direction of her life. For more than a year, she has had no-one to turn to, no-one with whom to share her pain. As a last, desperate act, she is seeking assistance and advice. She puts her objective bluntly: 'I want my life back'.

Such moral disorientation does not represent a psychiatric condition. Diedre is appropriately despondent about her illness. The fixed points in her world have been destroyed. She has been set adrift in an existential sense: she has no way of recognising what is of value to her, of establishing or ordering the things that are important. Her lifeworld—once vibrant and joyful—is characterised by uncertainty, fragility and precariousness. Ironically, although she feels that she was betrayed by medicine in the past, it is to medicine that she turns again. The problem arose in the clinic; she seeks to resolve it there too.

The task of a doctor here is clearly a complex one. He or she must analyse the patient's current physical status, make an assessment about the need for further treatment, and provide the information she seeks. More importantly, however, and indeed, as a precondition for success, it is necessary for the doctor to re-establish for her the credibility of medicine as a whole. He or she must engage her in a dialogue about her values and aspirations; he or she must stimulate a questioning about her body and its social and biological functioning. In this process, it is the dialogue that is important: the doctor cannot seek to direct or fashion her world according to his or her own plan. This does not mean that the task here is to re-establish 'autonomy' (as a bioethicist might put it), at least in a narrow sense: it is more about sharing responsibility. Nor is this a case of treating the 'whole' patient, as is sometimes said. On the contrary, the doctor has access to no more than a fragment of her life—that part that manifests itself within the horizons of the clinic. The doctor does not know 'who' she is, and, indeed, does not need to know. Nonetheless, the dialogue is not any ordinary dialogue: it is a therapeutic interchange that is rigorously structured in relation to the discursive forms of the clinic. As a therapeutic dialogue, it is directed towards making use of the destabilisation of her existing framework of values to provoke an enhanced self-understanding of both her predicament and the process of questioning itself.

Every individual inhabits a space of questions about what is good or bad, what is worth doing and what is not, what has meaning and importance and what is trivial or secondary[5]—that which is being called here a moral space. Within this region, decisions are made about contending values, about personal priorities and aspirations, about conflicting interests within relationships. Each person constructs a distinctive moral space of his or her own that acquires a sense of coherence and unity. The decision to take up landscape gardening, and the meaning of this activity; the experience of her body as youthful, vigorous and potent; the quality and significance of her personal relationships, including her relationships with her children; the impact of disease and pain and the imminent threat of death and disability—these components of Diedre's experience, among others, mark the structures of her moral space. This space forms a dimension of her personal life; it is a component of her lifeworld, that realm of immediate experience and face-to-face interactions. With her, as with others, conflicts may occur with people with different moral perspectives. Uncertainty and doubt can also develop, leading to internal conflict or a loss of moral orientation; sometimes both can reach pathological proportions.

The moral space is implicated in clinical medicine in several different ways. It substantially determines the manner of the interaction between doctor and patient; it provides the field of problems or issues that the clinical encounter must address; it contributes to choices that are made regarding the technical aspects of diagnosis and treatment. As in any relationship, the moral spaces of both parties are simultaneously implicated, although the interactions between them are controlled by the larger-scale structures of the clinical encounter.

The moral space encompasses a range of questions, problems, values and purposes. These may refer to a variety of contexts and philosophical perspectives. Although in an individual case there is a sense of coherence or unity, a characteristic 'moral style', this is not based on an a priori commitment to a particular concept of the good or of the good life. Rather, each person develops a set of values and a set of convictions regarding what is right or important: within the lifeworld, as has already been said, there is no concept of the good, but only multiple goods and values.

The notion of moral space is a version of the idea of moral identity appropriate for the contemporary cultural configuration. It places the moral orientation of an individual at the centre of his or her social interactions; indeed, it suggests that relationships only exist in the context of prior moral commitments. This formulation diverges from traditional views of moral identity, in which it is assumed that identities are stabilised around systems of fixed coordinates or universal principles. Indeed, the very notion of a sense of self in the classical accounts was dependent on a sense of the good. The self, or personal identity, provided the means for locating the subject in relation to established systems of belief and value: it defined the link with Reason, God, and History. In other words, as Zygmunt Bauman has put it,

> 'Identity' is the name given to the sought escape from … uncertainty … Identity is a critical projection of what is demanded and/or sought upon 'what is', with an added proviso that it is up to the 'what is' to rise, by its own effort, to the 'sought/demanded'; or, more exactly still, identity is an oblique assertion of the inadequacy or incompleteness of the 'what is'.[6]

The modern issue of identity was to keep it solid and stable. Under conditions of postmodernity, it is impossible to appeal to universal moral coordinates, and, indeed, this heterogeneity and pluralism is itself regarded as a value. Accordingly, the postmodern problem is just the opposite: it is how to avoid fixing the variables and how to keep the options open.[7] No longer can human identity be understood as a transcendence of the individuality and specificity of social and corporeal life. Indeed, it is recognised to be rooted in the present, inseparable from social life and dependent on the modalities of physical and sensory experience. This concept of identity was rendered necessary by the insight—supplied by Nietzsche and Freud at the height of the age of modernity—that it is impossible to understand the individual merely as a worker, consumer or even as a citizen. They showed (in the words of Alain Touraine) that the individual 'has ceased to be a purely social being and has become a being of desire inhabited by impersonal forces and languages, as well as an individual or private being'.[8]

In the moral lifeworld of the clinic, at the intimate level of the interchange between patient and caregiver, the patient confides his or her story, and the shape of the clinical consultation is fashioned and refashioned. Here, different moral styles compete, and a multiplicity of voices and experiences, ambivalent desires and uncertain choices contend. The moral space, in other words, is marked by 'heteroglossia': in the lived experience of the clinic, moral issues are shaped and individualised, and moral actors find themselves confronted with a 'multitude of routes, roads and paths ...'[9]

The moral space has been described as a region within the lifeworld. It is, however, possible to think of the lifeworld itself as inherently ethical in character. As discussed above, the most fundamental fact is the ethical relation, the quintessential encounter with otherness, with alterity. Ethics is the 'putting into question of my spontaneity by the presence of the other', which fixes the point of alterity.[10] The encounter with the other arises in the primordial relationship of the 'face to face relation', which well represents the clinical encounter. The face is the way in which the other presents himself or herself; the face-to-face relation is a confrontation that is open and unfettered but recognises irreducible difference.

It is not the job of the clinical encounter to reverse the disruption of Diedre's moral space, to restore some putative, pre-existing equilibrium. It is true that the exchanges around values in the interactive field of the clinic can alleviate anxieties or doubts, reassure or even stimulate processes of questioning. However, in this case, as in any other, the space between the patient and the doctor is marked by the irreducible fact of alterity. This adds to the clinical encounter an intractability and a perplexity that is a major source of its fecundity. The structured alterities of the clinic can provide the background against which Diedre can reconstitute her world of values and relationships. By resolving the technical issues, the clinical interaction can clarify the factual basis of her physical symptoms. Through this means, and through the process of the interaction itself, it can facilitate the deep interrogation that has to this point been obstructed.

The identity of an individual subject is secondary to alterity. Indeed, the other in a sense constitutes, and has priority over, the subject. It renders the latter open to others and it opens the world itself to the subject. Ethics is the domain of the response to the other's needs, and it is a responsibility for the other's actions—even if those actions are inflicted on the subject.[11] Herein lies another dimension to the complexity—and the potential richness—of the ethical relationship between Diedre and her physician. It is not the goal of the encounter to establish her autonomy, in the sense of specifying her ethical identity, any more than the existence of such autonomy can be taken as a premise; rather, in the process of the interaction itself, both confront and utilise the intractable and tantalising a priori fact of the autonomy of the other.

Motifs of Disruption

Emma is a 48-year-old woman who has been a successful actress and is now a promising painter. She is presently experiencing hormonal changes associated with menopause that are producing a variety of symptoms causing significant discomfort. She experiences hot flushes many times a day and she wakes, drenched in sweat, several times a night. She also complains of, among other things, extreme and debilitating tiredness and lethargy, unpredictable moods and outbursts of anger, and an abiding sense of emptiness.

She speaks eloquently about what she is going through. Her body, she says, is like a stranger to her now; it seems external, separate, a nuisance. Once she took it for granted; now she talks to it and asks it questions. Her world used to be organised, stable and predictable; now it is confused and chaotic. She was once celebrated for her savoir faire; today, she avoids other people because of her inability to control her impatience with them and her frequent explosions of anger. Her paintings have changed too: whereas five years ago she was painting large, brightly coloured canvases, today, the colours are muted, the mood is sombre and introverted, and the emphasis is on intricate, carefully executed patterns and designs.

She has an ongoing sexual relationship with a male friend, and this has suffered because of reduced sexual desire and difficulty reaching orgasm. However, she does not cite this as a matter of serious concern. Rather, it is for her just another symptom of the general malaise that has thrown her whole world into question.

One of the main components of the moral space to which medicine has access is the body. Of course, it is obvious that the body is, in some sense, the 'object' of medicine. However, it is not, as earlier medical ideologies tried to portray it, simply an inert object of scientific knowledge or therapeutic action. It is, rather, a complex social construction, deeply infused with questions of values. It is the source of meaning and meaning creation—and critical reflections on meaning itself. It is the perspective from which we enter the world.

The classical account of the body as the objectivistic target of medical technologies arises from the Cartesian tradition of medicine. Here, the corpse is granted epistemological primacy, and the living body is treated as essentially no more that an elaborate physiological and biochemical apparatus.[12] There can be no doubt that the Cartesian paradigm has yielded impressive results, including some of the most striking technical achievements of contemporary medicine. However, the price of this success was the omission of a vast field of meaning and experience, an omission that, at least in principle, imposes an internal limit on both the analytical and the therapeutic potentials of medicine. Medicine is, in fact, concerned with the body not simply as a physiological system, but as the site of lived experiences. This 'lived body', furthermore, cannot be understood merely as the objectivistic body with some additional conditions: rather, it is itself the condition underlying all conditions. As Merleau-Ponty once said, the body is 'the house we inhabit', the setting within which the world is revealed to us.

The concern of medicine with the manifold of embodied experience is not restricted to the general topography of the latter but extends to the ways in which it can be disrupted. In conditions of disease or illness, the body becomes experienced as a problematic or disharmonious thing, and therefore is in some fashion cast into doubt. An example may be given of the experience of pain, which has been analysed by Drew Leder. As Leder puts it, pain is 'ultimately a manner of being-in-the-world'. Occurring in a body previously free from it, it 'reorganises our lived space and time, our relations with others and with ourselves'[13]; it induces a split between our own sense of reality and the reality of other persons; and it causes a split between the mind and the body.[14] This applies equally to any other process that throws into question modes of bodily being formerly taken for granted, including disease in general, pregnancy, puberty, ageing and menopause. In all these cases, apparently unproblematic modes of corporeality are disrupted and the subject is led to a reflection on his or her bodily performance. In many cases, the transformation, which may be abrupt and unexpected, may be unsettling or even threatening; in some others, it may lead to a new closeness to, and an enhanced valuation of, the body.[15] There may be a sense of decay or loss, or, occasionally, even one of renewal or exhilaration. Leder's Heideggerian language aside, this description is consistent with Emma's experience: she too encountered a 'novel body' brought into existence through processes that subverted pre-existing assumptions, and that carried with it new internal spatial and temporal structures.[16]

The tendency to ignore the existential dimension of illness and to treat all physical disturbances as narrowly biological in nature has led to the disruptions that occur at the psychological, social or moral levels being largely obscured. Despite the widespread critiques of medicine, such 'reductionist' paradigms are now deeply embedded in the medical culture; indeed, they have become more firmly entrenched than ever with the success of new techniques in biological research such as molecular biology. In the context of menopause, biological reductionism—often referred to, inappropriately, as 'medicalisation'—manifests itself as a conflation of lived experience and the dominant discourses of disease and illness. It thus represents an annulment of the subversive potential of the physical disruptions associated with menopause, a rejection of any possibility that they might give rise to challenges to the constraining influences of ideology and culture.

The Cartesian tradition of a medicine that aims at the normalisation of the body is often opposed to the Christian one of redemption through suffering. Neither, however, adequately captures the complexity of, or the depth of meaning arising out of, the experience of the physical transformations that may occur through the life course. This point was made very forcefully by Friedrich Nietzsche, who trenchantly, and in characteristically grandiose terms, attacked both perspectives:

> [O]ur dear pitying friends ... wish to help [but] have no thought of the personal necessity of distress, although terrors, deprivations, impoverishments, midnights, adventures, risks, and blunders are as necessary for me and for you as are their opposites. It never occurs to them that, to put it mystically, the path to one's own heaven always leads through the voluptuousness of one's own hell ...[17]

The experiences of the motifs of disruption of menopause are extremely heterogeneous. As is shown by the case of Emma—and, indeed, the others discussed in this chapter—they are also highly idiosyncratic, varying with the nature and severity of the processes and contingent internal variables. From a clinical point of view, this means that few generalisations can be made, with even the commonest 'symptom' being experienced in widely varying ways. Nonetheless, it frequently occurs, no doubt as a result of the withdrawal of positive values attached to ageing at the cultural level and the devaluation of the postmenopausal woman at the social level, that the experiences of menopause become linked to images of deterioration and decay. Often, the raising of the issue of ageing provokes reflections on the question of mortality, undoubtedly made more poignant by the deep ambivalence of our culture towards death and dying. Menopause, ageing and death, disengaged from global social traditions that supply meaning and purpose, lose their coherence psychologically, and become precipitous and terrifying.[18]

To associate menopause with a narrow tendency to biological reductionism, or with a fear of ageing and death, may, in the contemporary climate, seem a pessimistic interpretation. After all, important changes have occurred, of which the present discussion itself is, at least in part, an outcome. There have been strenuous attempts to reverse and challenge at the cultural level the values attached to ageing and menopause; hence the proliferation of books with titles like *Journey through Menopause* and *Transformation through Menopause*. In addition, a greater, welcome openness about menopause has developed both in private conversation and in the public media. It is widely argued that women, being free subjects, should be able to make their own decisions about the issues affecting them and about the treatments to which they are to be subjected. The emphasis in the popular literature on women making their own decisions and on exercising their autonomy, however, does little to challenge the narrow conceptions of the body assumed by the dominant medical paradigms. Putting aside the obvious point that much of this literature merely reproduces uncritically the narrow biomedical perspective, the preoccupation with 'autonomy', as Rosalyn Diprose has shown[19], takes for granted that a woman's body is an object of exchange and regulation and that the question to be decided is just who should exercise sovereignty over it: the woman 'herself' (that is, considered separately from her body), the biomedical practitioner or perhaps the bioethicist (as representative of the law and the common good). The use—either explicit or implicit—of ethical 'principles', according to this argument, actually exacerbates the distancing of the agent from her body and from others, and contributes to the enforcement of a covert disciplinary regime. Behind the veil of universal principles and the liberal democratic pretext of enhancing the freedom of the menopausal woman, the reality is that the tendency to control the body and to ensure that it remains compliant and pliable—that is, compatible with the social body—is reinforced.

Medicine contributes to the maintenance of the disciplinary structures by means of which the bodies of individuals are in various ways organised, controlled and subjugated. These structures are very elaborate and draw on a variety of sources, ranging from the epistemologies of science to universalistic ethical theories. In spite of the complexity of this system of domination, however, the varieties of embodied experience can never be fully contained. They cannot be precisely delineated and organised around a set of principles, no matter how intricate. For this reason, the account given here is not a pessimistic one. As Emma herself shows, the body always retains an irreducible capacity for resistance and subversion.

Indeed, the category of the body itself is unpredictable and heterogeneous, and it is from this that the subversive capacity of embodiment derives. The category of the body embraces irreconcilable and incommensurable elements. There is no monolithic entity, 'the body'. There are only particular kinds of bodies.[20] There are anatomical and physiological bodies, male and female bodies, imaginary bodies, lived bodies, discursive bodies and poetic bodies. These bodies can be intertwined and contain social and cultural as well as physical attributes, and they may be disrupted and diseased. Furthermore, these disruptions themselves contain a subversive potential: they may actually expand experience and open up new possibilities. On occasions, because of the embeddedness of embodied experience in moral space, the process of disruption may challenge fundamental assumptions about meaning or values, thus further expanding and obscuring limits and boundaries.[21]

The Veil of Possibilities

Clinical space is complex and multilayered. It includes a variety of discourses deriving from the many facets of medicine on the one hand, and from the proliferation of the social formations of power on the other. It also embraces various discourses and voices coming from the women themselves.

I have argued that the clinical space of menopause is a moral space: it is a field of ferment, of negotiation and conflict over values. Like all spaces, real and metaphorical, it has boundaries. In this case, the boundaries are set by the horizons of the clinic itself and by the structures of the relationships that are possible under the general rubric of clinical medicine. These horizons and structures themselves depend upon different cultural and epistemological variables. This is due to both the large-scale social constructions that shape the clinical encounter, and the mutual nature of the relationship, which includes the doctor himself or herself—not just as a cipher of social discourses of power but as an embodied subject.

The intricate complexity of the clinical space is especially conspicuous in its ethical structures, which display certain fundamental divergences in comparison with the classical conceptions of ethics.[22] For example, as I have argued, given the diversification and differentiation of the project of ethics in the postmodern world, the field of ethical phenomena cannot be limited to the pursuit of the good life. Rather, evaluative activities that are not specifically orientated towards the good have become equally valid components of the ethical domain. Similarly, interactive behaviour with ethical content is not exhausted by theoretical discourse aimed at generating universally valid norms. While moral action may always carry some normative content, this may be only 'local', in the sense of being restricted to the immediate context of interaction rather than extending to the social group or the society as a whole.

Recognition of these basic facts may help us to understand the diversity and even contradictoriness of medicine in its intersections with complex fields of experience like menopause, and the ambivalence that develops in relation to it. It may make it possible to see how medicine itself can subserve a great variety of tasks and, at the same time, how menopause can manifest itself within its horizons in widely varying ways.

I have argued previously that medical practice—or rather the set of diverse, value-laden practices that constitute medicine—is, as I have sought to show, complex and heterogeneous, but nonetheless has a definite structure. I have in particular identified three strata that I have described in schematic terms as 'global', 'regional' and 'local'. The global structures are common to every interaction with ethical content and have the status of conditions of possibility of ethical discourse[23], and the regional structures comprise the ethical forms that derive from the social groups to which the participating individuals belong, encompassing the variety of social discourses. The main concern of this chapter has been with the third, or local, level, which encompasses the interactive practices that occur within the constraints of the lifeworld, or, more specifically, within the differentiated field of the moral space that I have sought to describe. This is the level of microethics—in functional terms, the substantive level of the ethical relationship, the field of face-to-face relationships, of local responsibility, of the meanings and values associated with sexuality and embodiment.

As pointed out, the three domains that constitute the ethical structure of medicine are interdependent. In any specific clinical interaction, all three levels operate to generate an elaborate moral configuration. This means that even those aspects of medicine that are, on the face of it, most straightforward can often be very complex. The cases of Emma, Carli, Diedre, Amelia and Brenda all at first sight involved only relatively simple technical questions. On closer analysis, however, a multiplicity of issues, each of great complexity and sedimented at different ethical and epistemological levels, revealed themselves. These issues cut across discursive boundaries; they embraced the biological, the social, the psychological, the existential, the sexual; they presupposed the existence of imperatives built into cultural systems as elaborate disciplinary structures, and the resistance to them.

In any individual case, all these factors may be visible at the one time. To illustrate this, I give the last word to the woman who, when considering whether to commence hormone treatment, expressed her misgivings with great power and poignancy:

> Why should I take hormonal therapy, with all its unknown side-effects, including possibly the increased risk of breast cancer, so that I will become dependent on my doctor and the whole medical machine just when I thought I was becoming rid of them, so that my husband will regard me as a 'triumph of science'—and merely in order to live for a few extra months, alone, when I'm eighty?

At the outset of this chapter I drew attention to a widely felt ambivalence towards medicine in the community. Among the things that I have hoped to show is that this ambivalence is not generated by either ignorance or ressentiment: rather, it is well founded in both the deep structures of medicine and the conditions that put people into contact with it. The clinical encounter is a site where conflicting themes and forces intersect in unpredictable and sometimes disturbing ways.

Like other domains of experience from time to time, menopause today has emerged as a battleground on which conflicts of various kinds—political, cultural, personal—are fought out. This means that many contending descriptions of it are available. Some of these defend medicine for its analytical capacities and technical potency, while others dismiss it for its complicity in the status quo. In a sense, all are right, since medicine is an ill-defined, heterogeneous collection of discourses, practices, tools and languages. Accordingly, both menopause and medicine can be sites for both affirmations of the existing order and for critical reflections on it; each can be a locus of moral action without defined end-points or unequivocal outcomes. This may seem a perplexing diagnosis on which to end, but in reality it merely repeats what on a larger scale has become fundamental for us. Indeed, as Nietzsche put it, perhaps this is the most powerful magic of life: it is covered by a veil interwoven with gold, a veil of beautiful possibilities, sparkling with promise, resistance, bashfulness, mockery, pity, and seduction ... [24]

Notes

1. See, for example, M Foucault, *The Birth of the Clinic* (London, Tavistock, 1973); I Illich, *Limits to Medicine* (London, Marion Boyars, 1976); J Ehrenreich, ed., *The Cultural Crisis of Modern Medicine* (London, Monthly Review Press, 1978); C Dreifus, *Seizing Our Bodies* (New York, Vintage, 1978); and many more recent examples.
2. PA Komesaroff, P Rothfield and J Daly, eds, *Reinterpreting Menopause* (New York, Routledge, 1997).
3. A Heller, 'The Contingent Person and the Existential Choice', The Philosophical Forum XXI, 1989–90 (1–2).
4. F Nietzsche, *The Gay Science*, tr. W Kaufmann (New York, Random House, 1974), p. 168.
5. C Taylor, *Sources of the Self* (Cambridge, MA, Harvard University Press, 1989), p. 28.
6. Z Bauman, *Life in Fragments: Essays in Postmodern Morality* (Oxford, Blackwells, 1995), p. 82.
7. ibid., p. 81.
8. A Touraine, *Critique of Modernity* (Oxford, Blackwell, 1995), p. 130.
9. MM Bakhtin, *The Dialogic Imagination: Four Essays* (Austin, University of Texas Press, 1991), pp. 276, 278.
10. E Levinas, *Totality and Infinity* (Pittsburgh, PA, Duquesne UP, 1969), p. 43.
11. E Grosz, *Sexual Subversions* (Sydney, Allen and Unwin, 1989), pp. 142–3.
12. D Leder, *The Body in Medical Thought and Practice*, (Dordrecht, Springer, 1992), pp. 17–37.
13. D Leder, *The Absent Body* (Chicago, University of Chicago Press, 1990), p. 73.
14. ibid., pp. 74, 77.
15. ibid., p. 90; see also S Gadow, 'Body and Self: A Dialectic', in V Kestenbaum, ed., *The Humanity of the Ill* (Knoxville, University of Tennessee Press, 1982), pp. 92–9.

16 See F Mackie, 'The Left Hand of the Goddess: The Silencing of Menopause as a Bodily Experience of Transition', in PA Komesaroff, P Rothfield and J Daly, eds, *Reinterpreting Menopause*, pp. 17–31.
17 F Nietzsche, *The Gay Science*, p. 269.
18 cf. M Heidegger, *Being and Time* (Oxford, Blackwell, 1978), pp. 179–85.
19 R Diprose, 'The Body Medical Ethics Forgets', in PA Komesaroff, *Troubled Bodies: Critical Perspectives on Postmodernism, Medical Ethics and the Body* (Melbourne, Melbourne University Press, 1995), chapter 10; and R Diprose, *The Bodies of Women: Ethics, Embodiment and Sexual Difference* (London, Routledge, 1994).
20 E Grosz, 'Notes towards a Corporeal Feminism', in *Australian Feminist Studies*, 5, 1987: 9.
21 'Even the determination of what is healthy for your body depends on your goal, your horizon, your impulses, your errors, and above all on the ideals and phantasms of your soul. Thus there are innumerable healths of the body; and the more we allow the weak and incomparable to raise its head again, and the more we abjure the dogma of the "equality of men", the more must the concept of a normal health, along with a normal diet and the normal course of an illness, be abandoned by medical men ...' (F Nietzsche, *The Gay Science*, p. 177).
22 See Chapter 1.
23 J Habermas, *Justification and Application: Remarks on Discourse Ethics* (Cambridge, MA, MIT Press, 1993), chapter 2.
24 F Nietzsche, *The Gay Science*, p. 272.

Part II

Love and Death

CHAPTER 6

The Many Faces of the Clinic

> O trees of life, when will your winter come?
> We're never single-minded, unperplexed,
> like migratory birds. Outstript and late,
> we suddenly thrust into the wind, and fall
> into unfeeling ponds. We comprehend
> flowering and fading simultaneously.
> And somewhere lions still roam, all unaware,
> in being magnificent, of any weakness.[1]

People go to doctors for many reasons: for the diagnosis and treatment of illnesses; to make sense of unusual experiences in their bodies that they suspect may be related to illness; for reassurance that they do not have a serious condition; for advice about how to avoid such conditions; for help in dealing with life crises like unemployment, bereavement or marriage breakdown; or for assistance with the passage through natural processes like pregnancy and menopause. Often, several such reasons occur together.

Take, for example, a patient, Rebecca, whom I have known for about ten years. Now a woman in her late fifties, she was born in Poland during World War II, where she suffered painful experiences that deeply affected the later course of her life. She came to Australia as a young child, married young, had two children and later separated from her husband. She worked as a teacher in country schools for many years and became quite a talented artist. In her early fifties she experienced menopausal symptoms that caused a degree of discomfort and anxiety that surprised her. Flushing occurred many times during the day and night, together with aches and pains, headaches, bloating and breast tenderness. She felt, she said, that her body was disintegrating, that it was out of control, possessed by a devil. She did not like going to doctors and was normally even less inclined to take medications. However, on this occasion she needed help. She needed assistance in keeping her body together and making her life bearable again.

Traditional accounts of medicine do not recognise the multifaceted intricacy and complexity of the clinical process. Since at least the mid-eighteenth century, medicine has been viewed as a singular discursive system, built around an epistemological theory of the body as an anatomical and later physiological and biochemical structure, unified by the methods and concepts of science. Even in more sophisticated recent accounts, which acknowledge the cultural contingency of the assumptions underlying modern medicine, medicine is considered to constitute a unitary discourse with a fixed concept of truth embedded in it. Ethical reflections on medicine have largely left these assumptions unquestioned. Finding the epistemological system to be limited to facticity, with no endogenous source of morality, they sought to append an ethical system, separated from the cultural sources that generated it, and subject to exogenous imperatives. In the appended morality, doctors and patients are invested with the capacity to choose between alternatives, to exercise their freedom, to protect and realise their human rights.

Clinical medicine, however, does not limit itself to a well-defined, rigorously delimited discourse of truth or morality. Rather, the encounter between patient and doctor—or, more generally, patient and carer—is highly heterogeneous and contingent on contextual features. The encounter is highly volatile and ambivalent, as any encounter between two embodied subjects must be. The clinical dialogue evokes and creates memories, causes and alleviates pain, disassembles and rejoins, dissembles and enjoins promises.

******

The patient's story never comes out as a single, coherent account. It is fluid, unpredictable and fecund. As Rebecca tells the story of her illness, she moves seamlessly between different kinds of language. There is the language of scientific medicine, of symptoms and causes—menopause, hormonal changes, hot flashes and arthralgias. There are experiential descriptions of their impact—the sense of decay, the palpable experience of mortality. There are also psychological reflections, philosophical meditations, sexual conflicts and challenges, the crystallisation of past experiences.

This heterogeneity is typical of clinical discourse. The language of science, which is directed towards mastery over mute objects, brute things, that do not reveal themselves in words, that do not comment on themselves, is only one among many in the clinic. Just as important are those discourses that seek to accomplish the task of establishing, transmitting and interpreting the meanings of the illness and of the scientific facts. In the clinic, and no doubt more widely, there is no unitary, singular or sacrosanct language. Rebecca can relay facts carefully and precisely, she can speak passionately and poetically of her feelings, or she can imagine and invent. Language is present only as something stratified and heteroglot.[2] This is not unlike the appearance of language in the novel, which also incorporates a diversity of speech types and voices. A single sentence can contain scientific jargon, colloquial language, language specific to age or ethnic groups, sometimes conveying social prejudice or political outlook.[3] It can convey precise scientific formulations or vague psychological speculations or deep philosophical reflections. All these linguistic and discursive modalities are specific points of view on the world, ways of conceptualising it in words, each characterised by its own objects, meanings and values. As such, they may be juxtaposed to one another, mutually supplement one another, contradict one another and be interrelated dialogically.[4]

Rebecca's attendance in the clinic, like her story and her language, is erratic and unpredictable. She sometimes disappears for months at a time, then returns or telephones, demanding the opportunity to talk and to be listened to. She cries, argues, shouts or just sits. When she talks, she mixes up facts and dates, and there are large gaps in her memory. She speaks about her current feelings, her relationships, her art. Most of all, she talks about her early life. As a small child, she spent three years in Auschwitz, where she experienced unutterable horrors, and both her parents died. After the liberation she came to Australia under the care of foster parents, whose relationship to her was never made clear. As it turned out, they were as scarred as she was, and she was subjected to terrifying ordeals in the new country, where it was never assumed that the family was safe from a repetition of the horrors of Nazism. Rebecca recounts experiences suggestive of much cruelty from her foster parents, though to be fair, the mutual pain was so profound that it is no doubt impossible to distinguish factual occurrences from fears and fantasies.

Rebecca's marriage was not a success and her relationships with her children were always contaminated by her wartime memories. She tried to establish a normal life and went to university and trained as an art teacher. This seemed to work for a time and she was able to maintain a job as a high school teacher for about ten years. She was evidently committed to her work and, it appears, well liked by her students. However, the inextinguishable memories of her early childhood repeatedly recurred and, once again, spoiled everything. She developed a range of symptoms—severe chest pain, arthritis, rashes, imagined cancers—that rendered her bedridden for long periods. She drifted between relationships, jobs, cities. She became a talented and successful artist, winning much praise and many prizes for her tortured and evocative depictions of the pathos and depravity of the human condition; however, she gave all the winnings away to charities, leaving herself in a constant state of poverty and privation.

******

The variability of linguistic usage in the clinical dialogue is not a purely technical matter: it is literally the means by which the patient reveals her 'self'. Classically, the self was conceived as a unified subject, in which being is homogeneous and indivisible. However, this conception of the self was just another manifestation of the universalising project in both epistemology and ethics of Western thought, which culminated in the European Enlightenment. The subject of classical philosophy was regarded as separated from the world, a solitary mind or ego from which truth appears to emanate. Modernity declared an identity between Being and Knowledge. 'The labour of thought wins out over the otherness of things.'[5]

Of course, this view of the subject was never uncontested, and it was pointed out again and again that there is a fundamental omission. As is demonstrated repeatedly in the daily experience of the clinic, the subject is not a unified entity but is radically pluralistic. It does not arise independently of social life or interpersonal experience. Subjectivity does not derive from a pre-formed cogito, or from language or society; it cannot be encompassed as merely an openness upon the world. Rather, it is generated out of the experience of otherness or, more precisely, the alterity between self and other.

The subject is strictly not a thing but a relation—between self and other, between subjects in formation, between 'intercorporeal' objects.[6] Similarly, truth is not an interrogation of sameness but an apprehension of difference, an attempt to grasp what is other. Reality itself is complex and heterogeneous, internally divided, a mixture of otherness and sameness. Our sense of exteriority, our inherent relationship to the world and other selves, is irreducible. There is 'a duality that concerns the very existing of the subject. Existing itself becomes double'.[7]

The many voices with which Rebecca speaks are authentic presentations of different facets of her self. She has occupied a variety of roles: as a victim of rape and torture, as a mother, an artist, a teacher. Like the language of the prose writer, her speech presents not only her different roles and experiences but also different strategies for engaging the world and other people:

> [C]ertain aspects of language directly ... express ... the semantic and expressive intentions of the author, others refract these intention[s]; the [author] does not meld completely with any of these words, but rather accents each of them in a particular way—humorously, ironically, parodically and so forth ... and there are, finally, those words that are completely denied any authorial intentions: the author does not express himself in them ... rather, he exhibits them as a unique speech-thing, they function for him as something completely reified.[8]

It is, therefore, not just the patient's language that is multifaceted and pluralistic: it is, in a sense, the patient herself, as she is formed and presented in the clinical dialogue. Her sense of physical decay, her overwhelming sense of isolation and loneliness, even the midst of large crowds, her fear of dying but lack of commitment to living, her inability to open herself up emotionally or sexually to another person—all these are not just symptoms and signs of a deeper, more essential, diagnosis, they are not mere epiphenomena: they are Rebecca's world of meaning and value; they are what constitutes Rebecca herself.

Her physical 'symptoms' too—the pains, the clouding of vision, the unsteadiness of gait and the falls, the conviction that she is suffering from an incurable cancer—are not merely incidental. They, too, are fundamentally constitutive of her world and fix not just its physical coordinates but also its values. Her body, like her sense of self, is the trajectory she traces out in her dealings with the world. Often, it is assumed by Rebecca's doctors that the illnesses she describes are either psychological in origin or purely imaginary. However, this is a mistake. Her pain, her symptoms, her lack of confidence in her body are certainly real. The hidden pathologies that so torment her body are the outcomes of the unhealed wounds sustained at Auschwitz, of the 'great death' within her—to use Rilke's words—that continues to '[hang] green, devoid of sweetness, like a fruit inside [her] that never ripens'.[9]

The body constitutes an axiological system: it is the site of meanings and values on the epistemological, ethical and aesthetic planes.[10] The values attached to the body are themselves subject to social processes and have undergone profound transformations throughout history. Since the Enlightenment, the body has been conceived as a self-contained entity wherein it 'degenerates at the end into an organism as the sum total of the needs of natural man'.[11] Illness involves a process of dissecting and reintegrating meanings of bodily experience. An important moment of the dynamic of the clinic is this process of revision and critique. The clinical space provides a setting within which this fundamental process can take place.[12]

******

Just as the patient utilises a range of discourses and speaks in multiple voices, so does the doctor. There is the language of science, of diagnosis and treatment; there are social and psychological discourses; there is interpretation, provocation, supportive dialogue and persuasion. But of fundamental and irreducible significance is the fact that the doctor is there at all, as a partner in dialogue. For not only do doctors and patients speak with many different voices, they speak to each other. In the clinical dialogue, the patient lays open her world, facing the mirror of alterity. In the controlled space of the clinic, she addresses herself to another person. She reveals herself for another, through another, and with the help of another. Only in this way, by a relationship towards another consciousness, 'by that which takes place on the boundary between one's own and someone else's consciousness, on the threshold', does she becomes conscious of herself.[13]

Dialogue is not an abstract linguistic exchange occurring between two pre-formed entities. The phenomenon of selfhood is constituted through the operation of a dense and conflicting network of discourses and signifying practices that are themselves bound up with the intricate phenomenology of the self–other relation. As Bakhtin put it, 'dialogue ... is not the threshold to action, it is the action itself. In dialogue a person not only shows himself outwardly, but he becomes for the first time that which he is ... not only for others but for himself as well. To be means to communicate dialogically. When dialogue ends, everything ends'.[14]

In responding to the call of the other, I Rebecca's doctor divest myself of intentionality and rational calculation. This is because in the crucible of alterity—and this applies equally to both partners in the dialogue—the self 'has no name, no situation, no status. It has a presence afraid of presence, afraid of the insistence of the identical ego, stripped of all qualities'.[15] In its nakedness, 'in its mortality, the face before me summons me, calls for me, begs for me, as if the invisible death that must be faced by the Other, pure otherness, separated, in some way, from any whole, were my business'.[16] In the pre-reflective proximity to another person, I myself am stripped bare; my 'ego (is stripped) of its pride and the dominating imperialism characteristic of it'.[17]

The starting point for meaning, value and truth is the face-to-face confrontation with another.[18] It is not subjectivity but the complex and pluralistic ethical bond to alterity that is prior. The experience of the other is over and beyond Being and its truth.

'The prophetic word responds to the epiphany of the face ... [T]he epiphany of the face ... attests the presence of the third party, the whole of humanity in the eyes that look at me.'[19]

It is impossible not to be drawn into the dark poignancy of Rebecca's world. In her cries—and in her art—she calls for witness to her suffering. All her life she has been a hostage to what has been called the age of atrocity. By becoming her witness one becomes her hostage, one's body aches while standing before her, bearing the guilt we all share for the monstrosities so many have endured.

> Before the neighbour I am summoned and do not just appear ... [T]he stony core of my substance is dislodged ... [I]n calling upon me as someone accused who cannot reject the accusation, it obliges me as someone unreplaceable and unique, someone chosen ... I cannot evade the face of the other, naked and without resources ... I am pledged to [her] without being able to take back my pledge.[20]

To witness suffering is a complex thing. It is impossible not to be drawn into it, even if, as a doctor, one has seen many people immersed in suffering. It is often said of doctors that they become hard and calloused as a defensive measure, to protect themselves. It seems unlikely that it is ever possible to become fully hardened to another's pain, to escape—as Hannah Arendt put it—'the animal pity by which all normal men are affected in the presence of physical suffering'.[21] The experience of coming into contact with suffering is described by Alphonso Lingis:

> We do not simply see the pallid surfaces, the contorted hands and fingers; we feel a depth of pain ... There is contagion of misery. For one does not view the pain behind the surfaces of his skin; one feels it troubling one's look, one feels it up against oneself. The sense of sharing the pain of another, the sense of the barriers of identity, individuality, and solitude breaking down hold us. There is anonymity but also communion in suffering. One suffers as anyone suffers, as all that lives suffers ...[22]

This does not mean that the clinical dialogue should be understood fundamentally as an expression of empathy, arising out of a relationship of reciprocity. A doctor does not provide support by expressing empathy or by establishing friendship: indeed, such relationships actually undermine the possibility of precipitating critical reflection within the many different kinds of discourse inhabiting the clinic.

The premise of anyone going to a doctor is that someone will listen to his or her story. The first act of the clinical encounter is the primordial first-person singular utterance, 'Here I am', which is heard and, like an outstretched arm, responded to by another.[23] The declaration is not an abstract act of self-positing. It presupposes alterity and the existence of the other. Thus, the face-to-face confrontation is not a relationship as ordinarily conceived: it is asymmetrical and non-reciprocal. The otherness of the other is irreducible and unfathomable. It is not reciprocal because humans are not interchangeable, or able to be substituted for each other[24], but it does entail an act of self-exposure and vulnerability.

> To be means to communicate. Absolute death (non-being) is the state of being unheard, unrecognised, unremembered. To be means to be for another, and through the other, for oneself. A person has no internal sovereign territory, he is wholly and always on the boundary; looking inside himself, he looks into the eyes of another or with the eyes of another.[25]

The clinical space is the space of face-to-face confrontation, of the subtle and irreversible play of alterity. It is also, of course, the space of language: after all, the face to face founds language.[26] But language is not just a vehicle for transmission of meaning, an untroubled promoter of communication, for it is the conditions for communication that are at stake. 'Saying is communication, to be sure, but as a condition for all communication, as exposure.'[27] Nor is it merely a medium for the play of ideas: it is the incarnate movement of the ideas themselves. 'Meaning is the face of the Other, and all recourse to words takes place already within the primordial face to face of language.'[28]

******

Both doctor and patient are in their own ways witnesses to suffering. There are two meanings of the word 'witness', which, as Agamben has pointed out, correspond to the two Latin words *superstes* and *testis*.[29] The former sense refers to 'the survivor', the bearer of an experience, the one who has lived through it from beginning to end, and has acquired knowledge about it from the inside, so to speak. It is in this sense that Rebecca—the patient—is a witness. The latter refers to the person who, in a trial or lawsuit between two parties, is in a position of a third party. This is the position in which I—the doctor—stand: as the one who observes, who sees from the outside, who observes and records the suffering.

The doctor hears and records the patient's experiences. He constitutes an active memory of them[30], an 'archive' of events, of experiences, of suffering. Thereby, he becomes a kind of timekeeper, a custodian of the past and one who defines the possibilities that might be realised in the future. His job, or part of it, is to assist the witness—the *superstes*—to integrate his or her experiences into a larger whole, and to pass them back to the accumulated knowledge and wisdom of the community. As an archivist, in this Foucauldian sense, therefore, the doctor does not just accumulate facts or propositions, symptoms and signs, dates, times and laboratory results. He assists the patient, often slowly, painstakingly, to construct a 'history', to define the conditions of the system of statements that constitutes the sum of his or her experience.

The archive that is constructed through the clinical dialogue is not an undifferentiated mass of statements that 'unifies everything that has been said in the great, confused murmur of a discourse'. Rather, it is a dynamic, reflective 'system that governs the appearance of statements as unique events', which 'differentiates discourses in their multiple existence and specifies them in their own duration'[31]; that is, the clinical archive recognises the multiple voices of the clinic and seeks to provide them with a topographic schema within which they can preserve their distinctive character, but nevertheless engage each other in a kind of internal dialogue. Thus, the medical diagnosis, like the archaeological one, does not establish the fact of our identity by the play of distinctions. It establishes that we are different, that our reason is the difference of discourse, our history the difference of times, our selves the difference of masks. That difference, far from being the forgotten and recovered origin, is this dispersion that we are and make.[32]

The act of witnessing and of creating the archive is a process of interpreting the traces, the inscriptions, laid down within Rebecca's body, both of the horrors of the twentieth century and of her more mundane experiences[33], of unjumbling her multiple voices, and of interpreting them, or at least seeking a place for them within a dynamic whole.

******

Over time, Rebecca's symptoms have increased and became more debilitating, and she has come to believe that she harbours a malignant tumour. A visit to the doctor has become a fearful experience, even if she also finds it affirming and comforting. She rarely keeps appointments, but when she does she will talk about her symptoms and her presumed illnesses at great length and with great intensity. In spite of this, she refuses to undergo tests, in the fear that the diagnosis would be proved right—or perhaps because it would be proved wrong.

The pain and other symptoms are undoubtedly both physical and psychic. Rebecca's appeals to her doctors for help are in a sense calls to heal the unhealable, the deep scars opened up in our civilisation by the abominations of the century just ended. But her pain is more than a metaphor; it is real, incarnate, physical suffering. Her pain reflects the anguish that has characterised almost every moment of her life, together with an underlying physical process, the nature of which at this time remains undetermined. Her symptoms cannot be understood either as merely psychic phenomena or as the effects of a biological process—they are both together: one gives meaning to, and provides the framework for, the other.

For Rebecca, every confrontation with a doctor is almost as challenging as the illness itself. In them, all her fears and hopes are crystallised, to a point that has become almost unbearable. On the one hand, she sees the prospect of a relationship of caring with another person who would assume responsibility for her welfare and in whom she could place her trust, a relationship that has evaded her throughout her life—a relationship that could, perhaps, in a limited way, make up for the chasm opened up when her parents were murdered before her eyes. On the other hand, the very same relationship carries with it the possibility of the pronouncement of her own death sentence, the confirmation of her terminal diagnosis. She understands that the moment of trust is also a potential moment of truth, and betrayal. Thus, the clinical encounter contains a promise, a challenge and a threat, all of which she well recognises.

Rebecca's ambivalent relationship to the medical profession draws attention to another aspect of the confrontation between the partners in the clinical relationship, one that plays a critical role in its dynamics: its potentially disruptive and menacing quality. Illness is experienced as a perturbing force, often dark and threatening. The exposure of the experience of illness in the clinic always, therefore, has a potentially disturbing, disruptive aspect to it. This is one of the sources of the peculiar power of clinical medicine: by addressing the patient as a singular being, by engaging her in her specificity, it can gain access to the most intimate recesses of that person's being. It can challenge meanings, undermine assumptions and provoke fundamental reassessments and revaluations.

The confrontation between the partners in the clinical encounter is irreducible; the moral exigency to which alterity gives rise is unsatisfiable. The other person cannot be thematised, objectified or totally defined. He or she is ambiguous, irreducible, infinite—infinitely transcendent, infinitely foreign.[34] The face is present in its refusal to be contained. This is the obverse side of the ethical relationship that subtends discourse: it is threatening and challenging, 'it puts the I in question'.[35] The clinical relationship is not just one of support and affirmation, but also of subversion and confrontation. Its processes involve not just the integration of experience, but disintegration, critical questioning, anatomising.

As mentioned previously, the institutions of totality can only judge the individual as a universal 'I', as the instantiation of a universal rule. Others as marginal—as face-to-face interlocutors—do not have a place. In contrast to totality, which always speaks in the third person, singularity speaks in the first person: it always has a name. When one comes face to face with another person in his or her singularity, one is exposed to his or her powers, and is vulnerable to his or her strength; but at the same time, one resists that power by calling it into question.[36] Through this mutual resistance and vulnerability, each party is challenged in a manner that is both threatening and affirming; each is called upon, 'to take the bread out of [his] own mouth', as Levinas puts it, 'to nourish the hunger of another with [his] own fasting'.[37]

Usually, this obduracy, this unsettling character of the clinical interaction, is not a deficiency. Rather, it is one of its greatest strengths. By calling into question the equilibrium formerly considered unshakeable—indeed, not even recognised as an equilibrium—by challenging the economy of the body, the possibility of new experiences and new meanings is evoked. The clinic is often the site for creative change. Illness, even supposedly trivial illness, can release powerful processes of meaning creation or rearrangement, of insight and reflection.

******

Alterity, the irreducible contact with otherness, is the engine of the clinical discourse. Despite its fundamental role, its boundaries remain indistinct. This is because the relationship between self and other cannot be formalised or subsumed under universal principles, since this would undermine its spontaneous, local character. Alterity simply is: it is a relation of pure immediacy. The mutual commitment of two people is a presupposition of all dialogue. In a sense, therefore, the other person is always already present within my self.

My relationship with another person is at once a relationship through language and through the body. Conversely, my experience of my own body presupposes my relationships with other people. For my body is made of the same flesh as the world, as Merleau-Ponty said[38], and this flesh of my body is shared by the world and by other people. There is, therefore, no brute otherness, and no brute world. There is 'only an elaborated world; there is no intermundane space, there is only a signification "world"'.[39]

As a doctor, I do not grasp the patient so as to dominate her; rather, I respond to her as if to a summons that cannot be ignored. 'In the exposure to wounds and outrages, in the feeling proper to responsibility, the oneself is provoked as irreplaceable, as devoted to the others, without being able to resign, and thus as incarnated in order to offer itself, to suffer and to give.'[40] The relationship with alterity is finding oneself under a bond, commanded, contested, having to answer to another for what one does and for what one is. It is finding oneself addressed, appealed to, 'having to answer for the wants of another and supply for his distress …'

> To acknowledge the imperative force of another is to put oneself in his place, to answer to his need, 'to give to the other the bread from one's own mouth.' On the other hand, [t]o put oneself in the place of another is also to answer for his deeds and misdeeds, to bear the burden of his persecution, to endure and answer for it …[41]

Like all other relationships, the clinical relationship is immanently ethical. However, as this account shows, this ethical character cannot be explicated in terms of a formal prescriptive sets of norms or principles. The microethical contents are irreducibly dependent on the specific details of an individual's personal history and the present context of the clinical dialogue, as the latter manifests itself corporeally and through language. The moral bond is irresistible and irrevocable, but it is also intractable and unlimitable.

******

There is no dénouement to Rebecca's story—either happy or unhappy. Years have gone by and, despite hard-won insights, her pain persists. Despite the small victories, she still hurtles from one crisis to another, each as desperate as the last. Her drawings and her paintings continue to reflect the horror with which her life started, and will no doubt end.

She agreed to undergo testing for cancer, and came to accept that she was not, after all, about to die. She has been able to establish a rich and nurturing relationship with a new partner, though one not without ambivalence. She still hankers after the lost community and family of her parents, and her parents' parents. But in this, perhaps, she is not different from many other members of her generation.

Rebecca's story illustrates some fundamental points about clinical medicine. It shows that there is no single, unitary discourse characteristic of the clinic, but that rather the latter is the site of a multiplicity of conflicting and overlapping discourses. It emphasises that this heteroglossia is not just a peculiarity of language, but that it reflects the deep structure of selfhood as it is formed and presented in the clinical encounter. It reveals that this moment of marginality that produces both uncertainty and anxiety is in some ways the real source of the clinic's inventiveness and potency. In other words, it is the peculiar structure of alterity in the clinic that is responsible for the paradoxical fact that medicine embraces both caring and confrontation. It emphasises that the clinical encounter is inherently a moral relationship, but that the conditions of morality here are very different from those presupposed in classical ethical theory. Finally, as in Rilke's poem, 'never single-minded, unperplexed, like migratory birds', Rebecca and her story remain infinite, open to new meanings and new interpretations, always unfathomable, always unfinished.

Notes
1. RM Rilke, *Duino Elegies* (New York, WW Norton and Co., 1939), p. 41.
2. M Bakhtin, 'Discourse in the Novel', in M Holquist, ed., *The Dialogic Imagination: Four Essays* (Austin, University of Texas Press, 1992), p. 332.
3. ibid., p. 262.
4. ibid., pp. 270–2.
5. E Levinas, 'Ethics as First Philosophy', in S Hand, ed., *The Levinas Reader* (Oxford, Blackwell, 1989), p. 78.
6. cf. M Merleau-Ponty, *The Visible and the Invisible* (Evanston, Northwestern University Press, 1968), pp. 140–2.
7. E Levinas, 'Time and the Other', in S Hand, ed., *The Levinas Reader*, p. 53.
8. M Bakhtin, 'Discourse in the Novel', p. 299.
9. RM Rilke, *The Book of Hours* (Salzburg, Salzburg University, 1995), p. 90.
10. Bakhtin provides an account of the history of the axiological assessment of the body in his early essay 'Author and Hero in Aesthetic Activity', in M Bakhtin, *Art and Answerability: Early Philosophical Essays* (Austin, University of Texas Press, 1990), p. 254–6.
11. M Bakhtin, *Art and Answerability*, p. 58.
12. See Chapter 5.
13. 14 M Bakhtin, *Art and Answerability*, p. 252.
15. M Bakhtin, *Problems of Dostoevsky's Poetics* (Manchester, Manchester University Press, 1984), p. 252.
E Levinas, 'Ethics as First Philosophy', p. 81.
16. ibid., p. 83.
17. E Levinas, 'Substitution', in S Hand, ed., *The Levinas Reader*, p. 100.
18. E Levinas, *Otherwise Than Being or Beyond Essence* (The Hague, Martinus Nijhoff, 1981), pp. 18–19.
19. ibid., p. 213.

20 E Levinas, *Collected Philosophical Essays* (Dordrecht, Martinus Nijhoff, 1987), p. 167.
21 H Arendt, *Eichmann in Jerusalem: A Report on the Banality of Evil* (Harmondsworth, Penguin, 1977), p. 106.
22 A Lingis, *Dangerous Emotions* (Berkeley, University of California Press, 2000).
23 cf. RM Rilke, *Duino Elegies*, p. 65: 'Like an outstretched arm is my call. And its clutching, upwardly open hand is always before you as open for warding and warning, aloft there, Inapprehensible'.
24 E Levinas, *Totality and Infinity* (Pittsburgh, PA, Duquesne University Press, 1969), p. 298.
25 M Bakhtin, *Problems of Dostoevsky's Poetics*, p. 287.
26 E Levinas, *Totality and Infinity*, p. 207.
27 E Levinas, *Otherwise Than Being or Beyond Essence*, p. 48.
28 E Levinas, *Totality and Infinity*, p. 206.
29 G Agamben, *Remnants of Auschwitz: The Witness and the Archive* (New York, Zone Books, 1999), p. 17; see also M Bernard-Donals and R Glejzer, *Between Witness and Testimony: The Holocaust and the Limits of Representation* (New York, State University of New York Press, 2001).
30 G Agamben, *Remnants of Auschwitz*, pp. 143–4.
31 M Foucault, *The Archaeology of Knowledge* (London, Tavistock Publications, 1972), p. 129.
32 ibid., p. 131.
33 cf. J Derrida, *Archive Fever: A Freudian Impression*, tr. E Prenowitz (Chicago, University of Chicago Press, 1996), p. 26.
34 E Levinas, *Totality and Infinity*, p. 194.
35 ibid., p. 195.
36 ibid., p. 199.
37 E Levinas, *Otherwise Than Being or Beyond Essence*, p. 56.
38 M Merleau-Ponty, *The Visible and the Invisible*, p. 248.
39 ibid., p. 48.
40 E Levinas, 'Substitution', p. 95.
41 A Lingis, 'Translator's Introduction', in E Levinas, *Otherwise Than Being or Beyond Essence*, p. xxiii.

Chapter 7

The Experience of Evil

I am going to talk about evil. I am not going to discuss primarily the defining characteristics of evil deeds, or the causes of evil actions, or the psychology of evil people. Rather, I shall examine the nature of the experience of evil, what it is like to be a victim of unjust, unethical or wrong behaviour—to be at the receiving end, so to speak, of an ethical transgression. It is interesting that, in comparison to the psychology and motivation of the evil-doers themselves, the experience of evil has been relatively little discussed, in both philosophy or literature.

True, there is the suffering of Job, the madness of Ophelia, the desolation of Anna Karenina. We have Hecabe's cries, in Euripides' play, when she learns that her daughter Polyxena is to be sacrificed by the departing Greeks:

> My child! So many pains are here, I cannot tell
> Which one to ponder. If I turn my mind to this,
> That other one will not let me; and from that a third
> Agony again distract me, grief succeeding grief.[1]

And we have the prayer of Gretchen, after the death of her baby and the realisation that she has been used and discarded by Faust, whom she had loved and trusted:

> Who gauges
> How rages
> Pain in my marrow and bone?
> My poor heart's reaching,
> Quaking, beseeching,
> Thou knowest, thou alone!
> Wherever I go,
> Woe, woe, oh woe
> Rends my bosom apart!
> Scarce left alone,
> I moan, moan,
> And weep to break my heart.[2]

But overall, these are exceptions. We hear much more about the suffering of Raskolnikov than about the pain he inflicted on the family of Alena and Lizaveta Ivanovna; about the exploits of Agamemnon and Odysseus than about the people they enslaved and murdered; about Richard III than about Hastings, Buckingham and his countless other victims.

In this chapter, I shall try to examine the nature and implications of the experience of evil. I shall argue that such experiences are not exceptional events encountered only by the great and powerful, but constitute an important component of everyday life. In addition, I shall propose that—apparently paradoxically—evil is not wholly a bad thing, but plays a constructive and affirmative role in the stabilisation of meaning and values for all of us. Finally, I will argue that encounters with evil are part of the daily business of clinical medicine, and that doctors must learn how to listen to the voices of those who have experienced evil, to understand them and to assist them with the process of accommodating and learning from that experience.

******

As a doctor, I spend a great deal of my time listening to accounts of experiences of evil, some of which arise out of medicine itself and some out of ordinary daily life. Let me give you two examples. Rose, a patient of mine, was found to have a large tumour adjacent to her uterus and was told that it was most likely malignant. Naturally, she was shocked and dismayed, but accepted the need for urgent treatment, which would normally include removal of the uterus, fallopian tubes and ovaries. However, prior to her operation she repeatedly expressed her strong desire to avoid any unnecessary surgery. She emphasised—to her GP and to the surgeon—that she valued her reproductive organs and favoured the most conservative treatment possible. During the operation, it was found that the tumour was in fact benign, but the surgeon proceeded nonetheless to perform a full pelvic clearance. Years later, Rose has not been able to recover from the shock of this betrayal. The sense of abuse, transgression and dismemberment will not leave her. She continues to mourn the loss of her reproductive organs. She is unable to enjoy sexual relations with her husband, which had previously been important and satisfying. Repeated attempts to obtain an explanation from the surgeon have been unsuccessful. To try to find an answer, she has embarked on a lengthy process of litigation that has taken her to the point of bankruptcy.

Another patient, Hanan, whom I see often, matter-of-factly recounts years of abuse by her husband, who uses her as his sexual plaything. She is repeatedly insulted and humiliated by him. She feels that her body is not her own. He does not give her money or include her in financial decisions, even though they are wealthy. He does not notice or, at least, acknowledge her pain, even though she makes no attempt to hide it. Although she will say openly that she regards him as a man without compassion or moral scruples, for religious and financial reasons she cannot leave him. When he had a heart attack and required surgery, she dutifully nursed him back to health.

Evil Today

Evil is never far away from us. We see it on television every day, we hear about it on the radio and we read about it in the newspapers. The Holocaust and the Gulag are household words, as are Hiroshima, Vietnam, Bosnia-Herzegovina, Rwanda, Kosovo, Omagh County and the World Trade Center. We recall readily the sites of famous massacres, such as Mei Lay, Port Arthur, Munich, Lockerbie, Srebrenica and Beslan. We witness daily the results of the callous disregard of the lives and wellbeing of ordinary people in the pursuit of military, political or commercial interests: here, the examples are too numerous to mention. Evil is not, however, just a matter of spectacular events, of monstrous wickedness or the extremes of turpitude. Rather, evil is also close to us, in our own experiences and those of others.

The sheer scale of evil in the modern world and its allegedly mundane character have often enough given rise to despair and quietism. Those who had come through the Holocaust could never come to terms with the defencelessness of European society against atrocity. This was especially the case for those who were most steeped in that society's highest values. Thus, Theodor Adorno declared, with bitter resignation:

> All post-Auschwitz culture, including its urgent critique, is garbage ... Whoever pleads for the maintenance of the radically culpable and shabby culture becomes its accomplice, while the man who says no to culture is directly furthering the barbarism which our culture showed itself to be ... Not even silence gets us out of the circle. In silence we simply use the state of objective truth to rationalise our subjective incapacity, once more degrading truth into a lie.[3]

Contemporary discussions of evil demonstrate traces of such resignation. But they do more than this. By dealing with evil as an event that occurs only on a large and dramatic scale, in far-off countries, to people with different-coloured skins, they reduce it to no more than an abstract category, a theoretical idea, disconnected from our own lives and experiences. The mundaneness of atrocity in the modern world has become a device not only for assuaging our consciences, but also for affirming and consolidating values and practices that should be exposed to scrutiny. It has become a device for drowning out the silent expression of experiences of evil within our own communities.

Radical Evil and Ordinary Badness

Before I go on, I should say a few words about the term 'evil' itself. Traditionally, discussions about evil have occurred in two contexts: the religious and the ethical. The former has been concerned primarily to address the problem of how the world can contain evil if God is good and omnipotent. Over the millennia, many 'solutions' have been proposed, which I will not discuss, except to say that the concept of evil as privation, corruption or the perversion of something good has almost always been a theme. In such a view—perhaps given the most definitive formulation by St Augustine—evil does not have an independent existence but is always parasitic on good, which alone has substantial being.[4]

From the point of view of the ethical tradition, the problem has been primarily to define the nature of good and evil in order to render them recognisable and so to develop criteria for identifying good, right or just courses of action, or, in the strongest cases, for specifying normative algorithms or rules of action. From this perspective, the ontological problem of evil has seemed of less importance, although it has not been ignored completely.[5] Indeed, Kant himself, probably the greatest thinker in the Western traditions of ethics, in a late text concluded that there existed an 'insurmountable wickedness', a 'radical evil', in the heart of man, which can 'by no means [be] wipe[d] out'.[6]

These discussions are interesting and important. Here, however, I do not wish to address the questions of either the ontological essence of evil or the algorithms for right action. Rather, I am interested primarily in the details of the experience of evil as a mundane event by ordinary people in everyday life. I do not believe that the word 'evil' is too drastic in this context. Indeed, English gives us no alternative. Whereas in the Romantic languages, one refers simply to 'bad', or 'badness' (*malus, mal, maldad*), which takes in both the everyday sense of unethics and the grander usages of radical evil, in the Kantian sense, in English, there is no other general term for the opposite of ethics, justice or moral conduct. Furthermore, by drawing attention deliberately to the ethical content of daily life, I hope to contribute to a process of reviving the moral content that has become enclosed in the category of evil, and of rendering audible the voices within our own communities that have been drowned out by the terrible cacophony of distant atrocities.[7]

Ethics in the Everyday[8]

I have argued repeatedly in this book that the ethical topography of daily life arises out of the details of face-to-face interactions between individuals within shared lifeworlds of experience. These interactions occur within, and are in part shaped by, the broader frameworks of society generally and the specific cultural discourses that constitute it. Applied to medicine, this means that ethical decision-making occurs not in relation to conventionalised pre-formed categories, but as a sequence of small moments that one by one are often either barely discernable or completely inconspicuous to the participants. In any relationship that raises the possibility of practical action, we engage in a continuous process whereby we form and re-form our conduct during the course of a dynamic interaction. As the interaction proceeds, our microethical decisions arise and pass away, driven neither by our own needs nor by those of the other, but by the dialogue itself. Accordingly, ethical decision-making in the everyday does not occur only in elevated, rare circumstances where I find myself faced with a momentous dilemma arising out of a conflict between two global principles. It occurs in the mundane flow of daily life as I negotiate the myriad small and large interactions that make up the rich substance of my lifeworld experience.

In daily life, as in the clinic, ethical decisions are everywhere. They determine the texture of every communicative interaction. They include both the substance and the style of our face-to-face relationships. They embrace the words we use and the performative contexts within which we enact them. They encompass decisions made on the basis of conscious reflections and choices among alternatives, and decisions made intuitively, in the hot or cold flux of flesh-and-blood encounters with other people. Our ethical competence—as opposed to the more formal 'moral competence'[9]—is a skill that we deploy readily and implicitly, and which forms the gangue of our lifeworld interactions.

In the clinical setting, the ethical content does not start or finish with the interactions between doctor and patient. Rather, the entire experience of someone seeking assistance in relation to illness or fear of illness is replete with ethical content. This includes the first contact with the receptionist or nurse, the arrangement of seating in the waiting room, greetings and farewells, and the enduring reflections and reconstructions. Errors or lapses in these areas can be as painful as those within the consultation itself. A patient who is publicly humiliated by a receptionist may be as vulnerable, and suffer as deep and abiding a wound, as the one whose concerns regarding the risks of a particular drug therapy are peremptorily and derisively dismissed by the doctor confident of the potency of his science.

The importance of microethics does not mean that theories that do not focus exclusively on local contexts of interaction are invalid or irrelevant. Rather, it implies that they themselves must be seen in context. The global, regional and local structures of ethical experience articulate with each other, and together make up the congeries of diverse, value-laden practices from which our social and personal lives are composed.

The Problem of the 'Arrow of Ethics'

When we engage another person in an interchange that involves some degree of intimacy, as is the case in a large majority of medical interactions, we therefore enter into a field of values that is unbounded and indeterminate. We find ourselves not seeking unambiguous solutions to questions concerning the ethical validity of propositions, but negotiating trajectories of values within shared lifeworlds of experience. As I have said, we proceed incrementally, in infinitesimal steps, as, by trial and error, we explore the topography of this lifeworld.

However, this account raises a profound problem. If ethical action in the lifeworld depends only on local, contextual variables, how do we choose from among alternative possible courses of action? If we accept the truth of Zarathustra's assertion—'He, however, hath discovered himself who saith: This is *my* good and evil: therewith hath he silenced the mole and the dwarf, who say: "Good for all, evil for all."'[10]—are our decisions no more than arbitrary? If we give up grand narratives, the categorical imperative and universal norms of action, what criteria do we apply in practice? What is the ordering principle that allows one direction to be preferred over another in the flux of the ethically charged encounter between two people? What determines the 'arrow of ethics'?[11]

It was widely assumed in the classical traditions of ethics that one of the primary givens of human intercourse is that it contains an underlying imperative to act in a manner that is right, that we are all subject to imperatives to do good or to act morally, and that these can be described in terms of universal principles, such as a categorical imperative, a Golden Rule or a principle of utility. But if our microethical interactions do not respect such processes of universalisation, the foundation for such imperatives no longer exists.

This point was strongly made by Mikhail Bakhtin, who showed that such theoretical formulations of ethics

> [c]onceive ... the category of the ought as a category of theoretical consciousness, i.e. [they] theoreticise ... the ought, and, as a result, lose ... the individual act or deed. And yet the ought is precisely a category of the individual act; even more than that—it is a category of the individuality, of the uniqueness of a performed act, of its once-occurrent compellentness, of its historicity, of the impossibility to replace it with anything else or to provide a substitute for it. The universal validity of the imperative is substituted for its categoricalness, which can be thought of in a manner similar to the way theoretical truth is conceived.[12]

In the light of such criticisms, many attempts have been made to rescue the possibility of an ethical imperative rooted in the lifeworld, including by Kant himself. A contemporary argument is made by Alphonso Lingis, who seeks the sources of the arrow of ethics in our most immediate social and carnal experiences. Lingis claims that the imperative has direct, compelling, primordial quality. It is, he says, 'met with at once. Whenever we form a concept of something we find ourselves obliged to conceive content correctly. As soon as we set out to relate our concepts with one another, to reason, we find we are subject to the principles of right reason'. This does not mean, he points out immediately, that the imperative itself is a concept. Rather, 'it is a command that we conceptualise correctly. It is not a principle or a law or an order. It is a command that there be principles and that our thought represent order—or that we represent the unprincipled and the chaotic correctly'.[13] While it is true, he says, that 'the imperative for law is a pure and transcendental fact, prior to every explanation and every purpose'[14], specific contents must be worked out in relation to the infinite details of individual phenomena: '[t]he directives we find in the night, the elements, the home, the alien spaces, the carpentry of things, the halos and reflections of things, the faces of fellow humans, and death have to be described separately'.[15]

In other words, for Lingis, the imperative includes, but also exceeds, rational judgement; its true foundations lie deep within the lifeworld experiences:

> Immanual Kant is wrong to recognise only the intrinsic importance of the rational faculty in what we have to do. In caring for a brain-damaged child, we acknowledge the intrinsic importance of a child who will not accede to the use of reason. In snuffing out a smouldering cigarette, we acknowledge the intrinsic importance of the sequoia forest ... What has to be done requires attention to the concrete particularities of this situation, and the thinking that recognises what I have to do is ad hoc. Envisaging the situation in general terms may well suggest that the kind of action, and the kind of implements that resolved a similar situation, may work here. It may determine a certain kind of action to be necessary ...[16]
>
> It is the intrinsic importance of what had required action to conserve it, rescue it, or repair it that intruded with the imperative force, the urgency, of *what I had to do*. I come upon a cigarette smouldering in dry leaves in the sequoia forest. Someone, in cramps or panicking, is in danger of drowning, and I am the one who can swim. The someone later, or myself, to recast the situation as an action derived from principles falsifies it ...[17]

Moral Consciousness of Evil

In spite of these arguments, there would seem to be little evidence for the kind of immanent and abiding intuition of the good that would be required for an ethical imperative rooted in lifeworld experience. For such an imperative would have to take the form of a general rule, and, due to the mutability, indeterminacy and particularity of practical contexts, such rules, no matter how fine-tuned, cannot in principle ensure an appropriate application.[18] In addition, at the proximate level of the face-to-face interchange, access to high-order categorical abstractions to which Kant, and even Lingis, refer is simply not available. Indeed, it is notable that the examples the latter gives all appeal to a high order of abstraction—caring for a brain-damaged child, saving a forest from destruction, rescuing a drowning swimmer and so forth. But when my decisions refer rather to the choice of a word to ask an embarrassing question, or the expression to adopt when one has heard a new heart murmur or felt an enlarged liver for the first time, there is no general rule to which I in principle can appeal.

However, this does not mean that no distinctions are available at the level of the face-to-face lifeworld interaction that is the primary ethical event. On the contrary, I believe that there is indeed primordial moral consciousness, though not of the good but of its opposite or absence, of 'bad', or of 'evil'. This consciousness allows us to distinguish a category of possibilities that are conscionable from another category of possibilities that are not. What exists in the lifeworld is a distinction between the *territory of good* and the *territory of evil*. Within each, many choices are available, none necessarily more right than the other. The job is to distinguish the boundary surface between the two.

The existence of a primordial consciousness of evil is in fact well supported by the anthropological literature, which well documents the proliferation of symbols of evil in all cultures, including the most ancient. This is a subject that Paul Ricoeur presented in detail in his work *The Symbolism of Evil*. Ricoeur demonstrates how fundamental the awareness of evil and its related experiences—impurity, defilement, fear, dread—really are. From his empirical analysis, he argues that in earlier societies, physical suffering was indistinguishable from evil and sin. The two were dissociated only through a massive work of culture, 'in the crisis of which the Babylonian Job and the Hebrew Job were the admirable witnesses'.[19] This dissociation, furthermore, became one of the greatest sources of anguish for the human conscience, for suffering has had to become absurd and scandalous in order that sin might acquire its strictly spiritual meaning. 'Man enters into the ethical world', he concludes, 'not through love [but] though fear …'[20]

What constitutes this primordial experience of evil? Here, some useful insights are provided by Heidegger and Levinas. In *Being and Time*, Heidegger analysed a common experience that he referred to as *angst*, usually translated as 'anguish', 'anxiety' or sometimes 'dread'.[21] Anguish is the experience of the weird or the uncanny, according to which we are removed from our concern about what is happening around us, and are led instead to reflect upon our own existence. It is the experience of finitude, of contingency, of the fragility of the conditions of the context of meaning in relation to which we orient ourselves.

Anguish, Heidegger says, 'reveals the nothing'.[22] We 'hover' in anguish; it 'induces the slipping away of beings as a whole'; it 'robs us of speech …'[23] 'In the clear night of the nothing of anxiety the original openness of beings as such arises: that they are beings—and not nothing…'[24] Through the disruption, the implicit threat, inherent in the experience of anguish, we recognise that we are thrown into this world, and are brought face to face with this thrownness.

Almost as an aside, Heidegger adds, paradoxically, that evil has an affirmative moment. It is involved in the conduct of 'historical eksistence, that is, the *humanitas* of *homo humanus*, into the realm of the upsurge of the healing …'[25]

> With healing, evil appears all the more in the lighting of Being. The essence of evil does not consist in the mere baseness of human action but rather in the malice of rage. Both of these, however, healing and the raging, can essentially occur only in Being, insofar as Being itself is what is contested. In it is concealed the essential provenance of nihilation. What nihilates illuminates itself as the negative.[26]

This is paradoxical because what is affirmed is the limits of human action and experience; that is, negation itself.

Levinas takes up a similar description in his own analysis of suffering and makes the direct link to the experience of evil. Considering the interpretation of the suffering of Job by Philippe Nemo, and in agreement with Heidegger, he interprets anguish 'as an unveiling of nothingness, as being-unto-death'. In the face of anguish, he says, 'the world slips away and isolates man, and man closes himself to words of consolation which still belong to the resources of the world that is coming undone'.[27] Anguish 'is the sharp point at the heart of evil. A malady, a disease of living flesh, ageing, corruptible; a declining and a rotting …'[28]

> Evil is not excess because suffering can be strong and thus go far beyond what is bearable. The rupture with the normal and the normative, with order, with synthesis, with the world, already constitutes its qualitative essence. Suffering, as suffering, is but a concrete and quasi-sensible manifestation of the non-integratable, or the unjustifiable. The 'quality' of evil is this *non-integratableness* itself ... Evil is not only non-integratable, it is also the non-integratableness of the non-integratable. It is as if, opposed to synthesis ... were found the non-synthesizable, in the form of evil, as still more heterogeneous than any heterogeneity subject to the embrace of the formal, exposing heterogeneity in its very malignancy.[29]

This, then, is the quality of the experience of evil. It is the sense of subversion, of a disruption in the chain of being. It is the experience of threat—not of physical threat, but of a threat to the whole possibility of meaning. Evil reaches me as if it sought me, Levinas says: it strikes me 'as if there were an aim underlying the bad destiny that pursues me'.[30] My wound is in the sense of betrayal, or of confusion, or of disorientation, or of humiliation, or of dismemberment. The contact with evil cannot be accommodated into continuing experience, it cannot be explicated or contained in language. My experience is of profound rupture in the fabric of communication, of the fragility not just of community, but of morality as such.[31]

Evil is not the same as suffering in general, as, for example, from physical illness. Furthermore, not all pain is the result of evil. The burden of evil in the suffering of Job did not derive from his original misfortunes, but from the indifferent callousness of his 'friends', who rather than comforting him intensified his pain by accusing him of having in some way offended God. The anguish expressed in his poignant cry, 'Have pity on me, O ye me friends; for the hand of God has touched me. Why do you persecute me as God'[32], is the anguish of the experience of betrayal, not of physical illness, loss or natural calamity.

Evil does not reside in the fact that a woman suffers the pain of breast cancer. It lies in the fact that her husband of thirty-three years leaves her for another woman in the very week that the diagnosis is made. The pain is not made less by the fact that their relationship had been difficult from the beginning. She suffers, mainly alone, during her slow death, disorientated, despairing, unable to reconcile the betrayal of someone in whom she had once placed her trust.

Evil does not reside in the bruises of domestic violence. It resides in the viciousness of the blows that produced them—in the man who comes home drunk again and again, who is deaf to her cries and her pleadings, who cannot appreciate the effort she puts in to support the family, to pay the rent, to care for the children. It lies in her sense of hopelessness, of nowhere to go, when faced by the conspiracy of the priests in the church who refuse to listen to her and who call her a liar when she tells them what has happened. And it lies with her doctor, who also refuses to accept her word—and the evidence before his eyes—against that of her husband, a prominent and respected citizen.

Evil does not lie in the fact that the man has severe chest pain that could mean cancer or a heart attack, which could leave the family stranded and unprotected in a country they do not understand, where they cannot speak the language and where they have few friends and relatives. Evil resides in the peremptory command of the nurse who runs the emergency room to the wife to leave her husband's side because her presence and noisy lamentations are inconvenient and disruptive. And it resides in her sense that she is in free fall, alone, exposed and vulnerable in a society that values efficiency and order above the welfare of herself and of her children.

The Boundary of Sense

Evil marks one of the boundary surfaces between sense and nonsense. At any moment in an interactive context, there is a category of possibilities that are supportive of the conditions of dialogue itself, of the continuation of the face-to-face encounter, with its deep assumptions of trust and openness. And there is a category of possibilities that threaten to undermine this dialogue, to dissolve it, to challenge its conditions of existence. It is this latter category that we experience as evil at the level of the microexperiences of the lifeworld.

To refuse dialogue is to put at risk what is most fundamental, and most enduring. That is why evil represents the threat of dissolution, of the impossibility of all ethical intercourse. Interestingly, a very similar concept of evil was developed by Benedict Spinoza in his greatest work, the *Ethics*. This is brought out well in Deleuze's commentary on this book, in which he draws attention to the parallels between Spinoza's theses on evil and those of Nietzsche.

For Spinoza as for Nietzsche, there are no general categories of Good and Evil: there is only good and bad.

> The good is when a body directly compounds its relations with ours, and, with all or part of its power, increases ours …. [T]he bad is when a body decomposes our body's relation, although it still combines with our parts, but in ways that do not correspond to our essence, as when a poison breaks down the blood.[33]

In his letters on evil, he develops these ideas further, to restate the seventeenth-century thesis that 'evil is nothing'.[34] What is bad, he argues, 'should be conceived of as an intoxication, a poisoning, an indigestion—or even … as an intolerance or an allergy'. There is no *evil* (in itself), but there is that which is bad (for me).

> Those things are good which bring about the preservation of the relation of motion and rest the human body's parts have to one another; on the other hand, those things are bad which bring it about that the parts of the human body have a different relation of motion and rest to one another.[35]

An immediate corollary of this approach is that ethics—that is, the typology of immanent modes of existence—replaces morality, which always refers existence to transcendental values. Morality is the judgement of God, the system of judgement, whereas ethics deals with qualitative difference in the modes of existence.[36] More importantly, however, this also means that evil no more exists in the order of essences than it does in the order of relations. Just as it never consists in a relation, but only in a relation between relations, evil is never in a state or in an essence but is in a comparison of states that has no more validity than a comparison of essences.[37]

'The relationship where the I encounters the You is the original place and circumstance of the ethical coming.'[38] A condition of dialogue is the non-indifference of the you to the I, which is itself a condition of the mutual self-constitution of identity that is implicit in all intimate interactions.[39] 'Dialogue is thus not merely a way of speaking. Its significance has a general reach. It is transcendence ... Transcendence has no meaning except by way of an I saying You.'[40]

The threat of evil is of ultimate chaos, of meaninglessness. Evil is the threat of imminent decomposition, of the dissolution of being, at the level of the lifeworld of experiences. It is the threat to the existence of ethics as such.

The Limits and the Possibility of Meaning

It is precisely in this contact with the boundaries of meaning that the positive aspect of the experience evil lies, and which constitutes one of the most important tasks of those involved in clinical medicine. Evil takes us to the limits. In experiencing evil we explore boundaries and thus encounter the possibility of new insights. The experience of evil is the experience of the edge of infinity, or the abyss. The limits of meaning are also the possibility of new meaning.

Medicine is a practice of meaning. It works at the edges of experience—the meaning of illness, the modalities of the body and sexuality, the power of suffering. It also often involves close encounters with the limits of sense in the form of evil, whether this occurs in the course of the medical interactions themselves or arises out of prior, independent experiences. Evil marks out the limits of understanding and intelligibility. We try to keep just on this side of the boundary.

The doctor's task is always to assist in giving expression to, and facilitating, understanding of silent voices. This includes the use of the experience of illness and suffering to generate new meanings. This is a dialogical activity that originates in a relationship. It is multifaceted and heteroglossic.

I have argued in this chapter for three main hypotheses. First, evil is not an exceptional phenomenon. It is an inherent feature of everyday life. The experience of evil is an important constituent of meaning and the locus of the absence of meaning. ('Evil is everywhere'.) Second, evil is indeed more fundamental than good. There is no imperative to do good. In fact, we have no specific criteria for recognising what is good, and many paths that we regard as ethically satisfactory. Instead, what we have is an ability to recognise evil. And third, the experience of evil has stable, recognisable features. We can identify characteristics of evil in the face-to-face setting.

There is an ethical injunction that comes out of this, specifically related to the task of medicine—and maybe to the tasks of other professions as well. The job of the doctor is precisely to listen to silent voices—to the painful experiences of ordinary people. Doctors hear about evil everyday—evil concerning relationships with partners and families, with government departments and other forms of authority, and with doctors and the medical system. One of our main tasks is to assist people in accommodating these experiences, in resolving the issues raised by them, and in enhancing their experiences of meaning in a more general sense.

Notes

1. Euripides, *Hecabe, in Medea and Other Plays*, tr. P Vellacott (Harmondsworth, Penguin Books, 1963), p. 80.
2. Goethe, *Faust*, tr. W Arndt (New York, Norton Critical Edition, 2000), p. 88.
3. T Adorno, *Negative Dialectics*, tr. EB Ashton (London, Polity Press, 2007), p. 367.
4. Augustine, *Saint Augustine: His Enchiridion to Laurence* (London, Thomas Clarke, 1607), chapter 4: 'Nothing evil exists in itself, but only as an evil aspect of some actual entity'.
5. See also AO Rorty, ed., *The Many Faces of Evil: Historical Perspectives* (New York, Routledge, 2001).
6. I Kant, *Religion Within the Limits of Reason Alone* (UK, Cambridge University Press, 1988), p. 66.
7. F Nietzsche introduced the distinction between Evil as a regulatory category linked to ressentiment by the Judeo-Christian tradition, a phenomenon of the 'slave morality', and 'bad', which was the obverse of nobility and goodness in the 'master morality'. See F Nietzsche, *Beyond Good and Evil*, tr. W Kaufman (New York, Vintage Books, 1967), passim.
8. See Chapters 1 and 2.
9. L Kohlberg, *The Philosophy of Moral Development: Moral Stages and the Idea of Justice* (San Francisco, Harper & Row, 1981), and J Habermas, 'Moral Development and Ego Identity', in Communication and the Evolution of Society, tr. T McCarthy (Boston, Beacon, 1979).
10. F Nietzsche, *Thus Spake Zarathustra* (New York, Modern Library, 1937), pp. 200–1.
11. F Nietzsche, *On the Genealogy of Morals*, tr. W Kaufman (New York, Vintage, 1969), pp. 36–40: '… in order to exist, slave morality always first needs a hostile external world; it needs, physiologically speaking, external stimuli in order to act at all—its action is fundamentally reaction …'

12 M Bakhtin, *Towards a Philosophy of the Act*, tr. V Liapunov (Austin, University of Texas Press, 1993), p. 25; cf. 'The categorical imperative determines the performed act as a universally valid law, but as a law that is devoid of a particular, positive content: law as such, in itself, or the idea of pure legality, i.e. legality itself is the content of law ....' (ibid., p. 25.)
13 A Lingis, *The Imperative* (Bloomington, Indiana University Press, 1998), p. 179.
14 ibid., p. 197.
15 ibid., p. 3.
16 ibid., p. 219–20.
17 ibid., p. 221.
18 MC Nussbaum, *The Fragility of Goodness: Luck and Ethics in Greek Tragedy and Philosophy* (Cambridge, Cambridge University Press, 1986), pp. 301–4.
19 P Ricoeur, *The Symbolism of Evil* (Boston, Beacon Press, 1967), p. 32.
20 ibid., p. 29.
21 M Heidegger, *Being and Time*, trs J Macquarie and E Robinson (Oxford, Basil Blackwell, 1978).
22 ibid., p. 104: 'The nothing reveals itself in anxiety ... Anxiety is no kind of grasping of the nothing. All the same. The nothing reveals itself in and through anxiety, although, to repeat, not in such a way that the nothing becomes manifest in our malaise quite apart from beings as a whole'.
23 M Heidegger, 'What is Metaphysics?', in M Heidegger, *Basic Writings*, ed. DF Krell (New York, Harper & Row, 1977), p. 103.
24 ibid., p. 105.
25 M Heidegger, 'Letter on Humanism', trs F Capuzzi and JG Gray, in M Heidegger, *Basic Writings*, p. 237. Dread is the uncanny awareness of the self to be either authentic or unauthentic, while the 'uncanny' refers to *unheimlich*: 'homelessness'.
26 ibid., p. 237.
27 E Levinas, *Of God Who Comes to Mind*, tr. B Bergo (Stanford, Stanford University Press, 1998), p. 126.
28 ibid., p. 127.
29 ibid., p. 128.
30 ibid., p. 129.
31 See Agnes Heller, *General Ethics* (Oxford, Blackwells, 1988), p. 170.
32 Job, 19: 20–22, in *The Soncino Chumash*, ed. A Cohen (New York, Soncino Press, 1947).
33 G Deleuze, *Spinoza: Practical Philosophy*, tr. R Hurley (San Francisco, City Lights Bookshop, 1988), p. 22. Indeed, all the phenomena that we group under the heading of evil, illness and death are of this type: bad encounters, poisoning, intoxication, relational decomposition.
34 See B Spinoza, *Correspondence*, tr. A Elwes (UK, Dover, 1951), pp. L31–38.
35 B Spinoza, *Ethics*, Volume IV, ed. and tr. E Curley (London, Penguin Books, 1996), p. 39, quoted by G Deleuze in *Spinoza*, p. 33, who comments: 'Every object whose relation agrees with mine (convenientia) will be called good; every object whose relation decomposes mine, even

      though it agrees with other relations, will be called bad (disconvenientia)'.
36 G Deleuze, *Spinoza*, p. 23.
37 ibid., p. 38.
38 E Levinas, *Of God Who Comes to Mind*, p. 147.
39 ibid.: 'Dialogue is the non-indifference of the you to the I, a dis-interested sentiment certainly capable of degenerating into hatred, but a chance for what we must … call love and resemblance in love … in the encounter, the other counts above all else. See also E Levinas, *Collected Philosophical Papers*, tr. A Lingis (Dordrecht, Martinus Nijhoff, 1987).
40 E Levinas, *Of God Who Comes to Mind*, p. 147.

CHAPTER 8
Death Sentence

Doctors have never been very good at dealing with dying. This is probably because dying is such a complicated business. After all, it's not just about diseases and medical treatments, but also society, philosophy, ethics and sometimes religion. The development of palliative care as a new discipline of medicine has provided important assistance to those involved in caring for dying people, and has generated a lot of knowledge about how to manage troublesome symptoms and various other medical issues.

Not surprisingly, ethical discussions have figured prominently in the development of palliative care, and consideration of ethical issues is now an accepted part of palliative care training programs and textbooks.[1] However, as with all practical skills, there's a limit to what can be learnt from a textbook. Ethics in particular is not something that can be categorised and summed up in a few rules or maxims: it has to be worked through—grappled with—again and again in relation to actual situations, with all their uncertainty and unpredictability. It's about negotiating values in complex settings, and its problems are resolved through communication and argument.[2]

To think through the ethical aspects of palliative care, it is necessary to try to understand what an individual goes through when he or she faces serious or terminal illness—to examine the intersections between, on the one hand, the powerful themes of health and illness, life and death, hope and despair, which are raised in such circumstances, and medicine and the caring professions on the other. It is necessary to follow the trajectory of a life, so to speak—with its problems and paradoxes, its accidental occurrences, its heroic and not-so-heroic decisions and their often unexpected outcomes—right to the end. That's what I want to try to do in this chapter.

I am going to recount the story of Maria, a patient who—however briefly—passed through palliative care, although she never came to terms with its premises or its methods. This is not the first time I have told this story, and it probably won't be the last. It is a story I find perplexing and, in some ways, disturbing—and this includes my own part in it. Let me start from the beginning.

******

Maria was just thirty when I first met her. Although I spent a lot of time with her, especially towards the end, there is much that I never found out about her, so I have had to try to reconstruct her life and personality from what others have told me. What I do know for sure is fairly mundane. She had been a teacher at a high school. Having studied classics at university, she taught languages and art history at an inner-city high school. At twenty-four, she had married Brian, a carpenter who some time later tried to set up his own business as a builder. Their relationship had been a stable and happy one. At twenty-eight she had given birth to Elena, who was the couple's consuming passion.

Maria first came to me in fairly mundane circumstances. She had a family history of heart disease—her father had died when she was only fourteen and an older brother just a bit later—and had been advised to seek advice about minimising the risk that she would die from this condition too. She in fact had quite high cholesterol levels and, after various unsuccessful attempts with diets, agreed to start taking some medications to try to bring them down—even though she always hated the idea of taking drugs. She was a confident young woman and an irregular attendee at the clinic. She was not universally liked by the clinic staff on account of her abrasive and demanding manner. Nonetheless, I got on well with her, possibly because I never contradicted her and never criticised her abrupt style or erratic behaviour.

When she was thirty-four, Maria was diagnosed with breast cancer. I wasn't involved in the diagnosis: she or her husband had noticed a lump in her breast and reported it to their family doctor, who immediately organised a biopsy that showed it to be malignant. She had the lump removed, together with the lymph nodes under her arm, one of which was found to be involved with tumour. A course of radiotherapy and chemotherapy was recommended in accordance with standard practice. It was in relation to this that Maria called me. She wanted to know two things: first, whether there was any chance that the medications I had prescribed could have contributed to the cancer, and secondly, whether I thought she should go ahead and have the adjuvant therapy.

On the first count, I told her that there had never been any link made between the medications she had been taking and cancer, so it was unlikely that the two were related in this case, though of course one can never be sure. Indeed, even though I have no evidence to support the possibility, as with other cases I've been involved in, I have never been able to dismiss the possibility that my treatments may in some way have contributed to her final demise.

On the second count, although I told her that it was established that additional therapy could reduce the risk of cancer recurrence, I didn't try vigorously to persuade her to undertake this treatment. I knew that she had always hated taking medications and that she considered them unnatural. She'd felt that even the anti-cholesterol tablets represented a significant compromise. I felt at the time that it was better to sympathise with her concerns rather than to contradict them, and that I should leave the decisions to her and her oncologist. In retrospect, knowing the final outcome, I'm not at all sure that this was the right course of action to take.

Even then I was struck by the change that had taken place in Maria. Her harsh and uncompromising exterior had vanished. Instead, she was scared—scared of suffering pain and of dying. The change in her circumstances had left her confused and disoriented. Her world had seemed so stable, her life so perfect, but in the few hours since diagnosis the stability had been shattered and instead of uncomplicated happiness, she was confronted with uncertainty and fear.

******

When faced directly, for the first time, with the possibility of death, Maria's moral world seemed to crumble. All that was valuable was threatened with dissolution. There was nothing left: no time, no future, no hope. This link between death and ethics is a natural one. Death, after all, marks off the boundaries of sense and meaning and therefore of value, and, in a sense, this is exactly what ethics also seeks to do. Death, like language itself, is the boundary surface between the known and the unknown, between coherent, stable communities of meaning and utter chaos.

We understand relatively little about the experiences of pain and suffering, and much less about the experience of death. There is no ready-made vocabulary to describe them. Of course, many writers and artists have tried to capture the experience, including the unpredictability and contingency of life. Kierkegaard warned that in the hidden recesses of happiness there dwells an anxious dread that is despair.[3] Dostoyevsky wrote of the experience of unavoidable destruction, 'the sense that a house is collapsing on you'.[4] Much earlier, Aeschylus had said that one could only know if one was happy at the last hour of one's life. One thing that was very clear in Maria's case, however, was that it was not a matter of personal happiness: it was one of ethical value. For Maria the question was the value of her own life, and the future for Brian and Elena.

Of course, being is never a purely individual phenomenon. This has been recognised by many philosophers. Emmanuel Levinas put it most bluntly, in what seemed like a radical inversion of the whole Enlightenment tradition of understanding of knowledge, the subject and ethics. Levinas argued that what came first was not the traditional categories of philosophy like 'being' and 'substance' and 'consciousness', but *ethics*—the elementary bond, the 'intertwining' (as Merleau-Ponty called it[5]) that joins people together, from which everything else follows. Indeed, individual subjects and the processes according to which we distinguish objects and construct truths, crystallise as secondary phenomena around this primary fact. It is, therefore, strictly wrong to call the ethical substance a 'bond' or a 'relationship', because this in itself implies the prior existence of two individual subjects who subsequently come into contact with each other, rather than being formed, constituted, crystallised, as poles of the ethical ambience. Nonetheless, the limitations of our language and tradition are such that it is extremely difficult to escape from these prejudices altogether.

Not only are our experiences of ourselves and others inherently ethical, they are also inherently *temporal*. What Western philosophers call 'subjects' or 'being' are in reality abstractions from every relationship with a future or a past.[6] Martin Heidegger—one of the thinkers who relied most heavily on the category of being—recognised that temporality is one of the fundamental conditions by which we recognise ourselves as individuals, either alone or in relation to others.[7] We experience ourselves not through contemplation but in the everyday acts of speaking, of communicating, with others, and this can only happen in time, relying on what has happened to create the new. The trajectory of an individual life is therefore a temporal phenomenon. We live in the present, constantly re-creating ourselves by continually running ahead to the future and drawing from the past. What exists for us now is like the tip of a welding torch, joining the past and the future. As Heidegger explains, in running ahead, our experiences become our future, in such a way that they come back to their past and present. Our experience is the experience of time itself, not something that happens *in* time.[8]

For Maria, as for us all, it was in time, in the possibility of a future, that she could establish and maintain her specificity, her individuality. Time is the source of our specificity, which can be maintained by running ahead to the certain yet indeterminate past. Human existence (or, as Heidegger puts it, 'being') always is in a manner of its possible temporal being. It is time, time is temporal, temporality:[9]

> … [T]he being of temporality signifies non-identical actuality. [It] is its past, it is its possibility in running ahead to this past. In this running ahead I am authentically time, I have time. Insofar as time is in each case mine, there are many times. Time itself is meaningless; time is temporal.[10]

Accordingly, the end of our own existence, our own death, is not some point at which a sequence of events suddenly breaks off, but a possibility which we know of in this or that way. It the most extreme possibility that we can seize and appropriate as standing before us. That which towers over every other statement of certainty and authenticity is the recognition of our own death, the indeterminate certainty of the possibility of our being at an end.[11]

******

Despite the issue with her father's and brother's early deaths, Maria's own death had always seemed very distant. Now, it was only too real. Work, leisure, the possibility of constructing the future—plans for the holidays, Elena's schooling, home renovations—all of a sudden were transformed. The pain—it was not yet physical pain—was very poignant.

Poignancy, of course, refers not to the experience of the sufferer but to that of the onlooker. It is impossible for a witness to suffering not to become engrossed in it, even if one has seen many people suffering in the past. There is no psychological or cultural panoply that can isolate us from the imploring gaze of the other. It is often assumed that doctors protect themselves from the pain of exposure to the suffering of their patients by becoming calloused and hardened. Such comments are probably based on a misunderstanding. Doctors do not offer support by expressing empathy or by establishing friendship: indeed, relationships of this sort undermine the possibility of precipitating critical reflection within the many different kinds of discourse inhabiting the clinic. But however this may be, it does seem unlikely that it is ever possible to become fully hardened to another's pain.

It is true that there are times, as when pain is heavily contaminated with power, when the pity spontaneously evoked in the presence of physical suffering is sharply diminished.[12] For example, in torture, the communicative exchange between sufferer and onlooker is lost: 'the prisoner's ground becomes increasingly physical and the torturer's increasingly verbal', so that the former becomes 'a colossal body with no voice' and the latter 'a colossal voice with no body'.[13] But—even if medicine itself is never entirely free of such contamination—this is an extreme case. In general, the onlooker—whether he or she be a friend or acquaintance, a professional adviser, or merely a spectator in the cinema—is drawn into the suffering:

One suffers as anyone suffers, as all that lives suffers. To look upon someone who is in pain is to have known pain, is to know what it is … One is repelled, but one is also drawn to that pain. The other is suffering a pain involuntarily; it awakens a will in oneself to suffer that pain. We cannot view the sufferer's contorted hands, his grimaces, hear his sighs and moans, without these inducing contortions, grimaces, sighs, and moans in us, and with them, inducing a sense of the pain. His pain, that pain that rivets the suffering one to himself, to the limits of his own existence, reverberates in us.[14]

One of the doctor's roles is to be a witness; that is, to record, to constitute an active memory—to construct an archive, so to speak, of the patient's experiences.[15] By so doing, he or she becomes a kind of timekeeper, a custodian of the past, and thus one who defines the possibilities that might be realised in the future. The doctor becomes a source, and a repository, of hope.[16]

******

After much agonising—and, no doubt, persuasion—Maria agreed to start chemotherapy, on the basis simply that it could get rid of the disease once and for all. However, from the very beginning she refused to put up with the side-effects and after only a week broke off treatment altogether. A few days later she telephoned me briefly to tell me that she and her family were the next day leaving to live in the country. It was only a brief conversation—I was busy and cut the conversation off short—but I remember it vividly.

She talked fast and her tone was flat and even. The chemotherapy, she said, just didn't feel right. It was out of sync with her body. It was trying to beat the cancer at its own game. You couldn't do it. The problem was, she said, that the assumptions of medicine were all wrong. Illness was not just a malfunctioning of a machine. It signified lack of balance, disharmony. Treatment had to re-establish equilibrium. Medicine wanted to control and organise everything, even death. If she was going to die, she didn't want just to be another statistic in the hospital register. She would die in her own way, in a manner of her own choosing.

She'd decided, she said, to stop treatment and to leave the city altogether. The whole family—I learnt much later that Brian had in fact been strongly opposed to the plan—was going to move to a remote part of the country to live on a commune where herbal treatments and meditation were practised. There, she would go about the business of healing herself.

As I said, it was a brief conversation, which I cut short. It had been just an ordinary day for me. I had a million things to do, mostly little things—phone calls to make, forms to fill out, that sort of thing. I was probably irritated by being interrupted and of facing the prospect of not getting away again till late. I said I was sorry I couldn't talk right away and asked her to call back later. I knew at that moment that I was making a mistake. She was calling to discuss a decision—that meant that she was looking for an opportunity to talk. This was surely a gap, a chance to change the course of events. If it was such a chance, however, it was one that was missed. Looking back, I have no doubt that this phone call was more important than all the tasks to which at that moment I gave higher priority. But I missed the chance and she didn't call back.

For Maria, a lot had happened in four weeks. But her story still had another two years to run.

******

Maria, of course was not the first person to question the conception of illness and death underlying Western medicine; nor was she the first to turn to alternative medicines to avoid what she regarded as the unacceptable side-effects of orthodox anti-cancer treatments. Indeed, the fact that the use of complementary medicines has become so widespread is an indication of at least a degree of disquiet about orthodox medicine.[17]

It's important to realise that the meaning of illness and death that today is widely taken for granted both within medicine and throughout the wider society is a historical and social accomplishment. Indeed, this is important for an understanding of the underlying purpose of palliative care, which addresses a problem that arose within medicine at a particular historical moment—the problem of the meaning of death within a culture that had mobilised itself to resist and deny death.

Much anthropological evidence supports the view that the concept of health prevalent in a society is determined by the dominant image of death.[18] Where death is regarded as a spiritual transition, illness is looked upon as a holy state; where death is a meaningless curse, the sick are not beatified but reviled and cursed.[19] In Western society, until modern times, death was looked upon as a natural constituent of life: indeed, killing the aged was common. This in turn led to a definition of health and wellbeing that was linked to a notion of a timely death. Accordingly, medicine, pragmatically, labelled people in two ways: those for whom cures could be attempted, and those who were beyond repair, such as lepers, cripples and the dying. The distinction between these two categories, and the recognition of the *facies hippocratica*, the signs of approaching death that indicated to the physician the point at which curative efforts had to be abandoned, was part of the medical tradition until the end of the nineteenth century.[20]

It is a widespread assumption in many, but not all, cultures that death is a process suffused with meaning. The exception is Western culture following the development of industrial society and the Enlightenment. There, death was transformed from an existential event into a mere natural object, capable of study—and ultimately, control—by the practitioners of medicine.[21] The power of this view of death in fact became almost irresistible so much so that wherever Western culture penetrated, its image of sickness and death followed. As Ivan Illich has pointed out, in retrospect, the suggestion that death can be understood and maybe conquered by science was an astounding—not to say risky—proposition, as Hamlet's uncertainty at the dawn of the modern era attests. Classically, medicine had not been able to conceive of itself as possessing either the knowledge or the insolence to oppose God's will. Indeed, it appears that the first mention of the possibility of the prolongation of life as a serious task for physicians did not occur until the time of Francis Bacon in the early seventeenth century.[22]

Gradually, new power was attributed to the doctor, even if there was as yet little evidence that he or she could actually exercise any influence over the course of disease. Death was turned from God's will into a natural phenomenon that could be observed and classified—and later, resisted or at least redirected. In a further transformation, it was converted into a mistake, an excess, an evil: an outcome of specific disease processes certified and—at least, potentially—controlled by a doctor.[23] This new entity was clinical death, which thus originated in the emerging professional consciousness of the scientifically trained doctor. Only after clinical sickness and clinical death had developed do we find the first pictures in which 'the doctor assumes the initiative and interposes himself between his patient and death'. In other words, it is 'now the doctor rather than the patient [who] struggles with death'.[24]

For many people—and Maria was among them—the development of medicine has therefore been associated with a shift in the understanding of death from something located uncertainly within the moral order to a mere phenomenon of the technical one.[25] Through the process of 'medicalisation'—as Illich called it—death and health care in general took the form of a technological system, bureaucratically organised and linked to social structures of power:

> Society, acting through the medical system, decides when and after what indignities and mutilations he shall die. The medicalisation of society has brought the epoch of natural death to an end. Western man has lost the right to preside at his act of dying. Health, or the autonomous power to cope, has been expropriated down to the last breath. Technical death has won its victory over dying. Mechanical death has conquered and destroyed all other deaths.[26]

Others have described the same process in slightly different terms. Ariès described the transition from a 'tame death'—that is, a death that was familiar, predictable, integrated into social life, recognised as subsisting within the natural order of things—to a 'wild death', which is an isolated or lonely death characterised by uncertainty, fear and degradation, the outcome of unfathomable and meaningless powers, such as those of technology and medicine.[27] Although these formulations may seem extreme, the point is nonetheless clear: the development of modern society and the medical culture that went with it converted death from what was primarily understood to be a meaningful process embedded in cultural structures and social rituals to an excess, a technical malfunction from which meaning had been extirpated.

******

It was precisely the gap between the moral and the technical orders, between meaning and science, that palliative care was devised to fill. Not that it saw itself in these terms, of course. Rather, the origins of palliative care in its modern form—which go back no further than the late 1960s with the opening by Cicely Saunders of St Christopher's Hospice in Sydenham, London—lay in a perceived need merely to care for the sick and dying. Coordinated medical, nursing and allied services were developed for people who were terminally ill, to be delivered where possible in the environment of the person's choice. Particular emphasis was placed on providing 'physical, psychological, emotional and spiritual support' both for patients and for their families and friends.[28] Thus, in place of the goals of 'curative' care, which aims at prolongation of life and survival, palliative care sought only to relieve symptoms and to ease the process of death. Whereas with curative care a high rate of treatment-related morbidity and toxicity was seen as acceptable, in the palliative setting, avoidance of toxicity and side-effects became ends in their own right. When death was imminent, all measures were withdrawn, except those required for the patient's 'comfort'.[29]

The moral specificity of palliative with respect to curative medicine derives largely from these discrepant goals, which also point to a certain irony in the history of medicine itself. Palliative care arose to fill the gap left when death was converted from a process loaded with meaning and spiritual significance to a mere fact of nature. The irony consists in the fact that, having created the hiatus, medicine sought to fill it by calling on the same technological and conceptual resources that had given rise to it in the first place. In this sense at least, the task of palliative care—to assuage the process of dying in modern society—was an impossible one from the beginning.

Maria's story, as it turned out, had an irony of its own. The family moved to their commune in the country, where they lived for nearly two years. They grew crops and made their own clothes. Maria adopted the philosophy and religion of Buddhism and engaged in regular meditation and other practices designed to achieve cleansing and healing. At the end of this time she remained well and considered herself cured. Eventually, the three of them returned to the city to resume their lives. I didn't see Maria during this period, and she didn't contact me. However, from time to time I saw references to her in the popular media. She'd became a celebrated figure within the alternative healing community and gave many public talks and interviews for newspapers and radio about how she'd 'conquered breast cancer without drugs'. She had become living proof of an alternative to the brutality of Western medicine and was widely quoted as a model to be followed.

******

But the story doesn't have a happy ending. Breast cancer is an insidious and unpredictable disease. About six months after her return, Maria suffered a recurrence. The tumour, now invading her bones, compressed the spinal cord, leaving her paralysed and without bladder, bowel and sexual function. Medical help was eventually sought but, although emergency radiotherapy was attempted, it was without effect. She was told that significant recovery was most unlikely and subsequently admitted to a hospice for ongoing care.

I went to see her the next day: I was unable to stay away. I found her lying quietly—sombre, calm, largely expressionless. When I came in, she lifted her eyes and smiled weakly. She sensed my unease, and no doubt the guilt I'd harboured since our last conversation. Perhaps to relieve me, she muttered that one of her aims had been to spend some good times with her husband and daughter and that she'd done that. Nonetheless, I was struck by an overwhelming sense of inertia, of resignation, that had replaced the intensity and determination I'd previously known.

It's impossible to know what kind of suffering a dying person is going through.[30] What is special and singular about death is its unsayability, its barrenness, its aloneness. The process of dying is truly a tragedy of solitude.[31] For this reason, dying—especially in pain and suffering—engenders a passivity and prostration. Death acts as a kind of sink for meaning, a black hole, to which everything tends but from which nothing returns. One is cut off from every living spring; there is no possibility of retreat.[32] This produces a kind of passivity, or prostration.[33] It also involves a unique, transformed, abrogated relationship with the future.[34]

As Heidegger has shown, death is the impossibility of running ahead, of having a project. The dying one endures a time without a future, a time from which the resources of the past are irrelevant and disconnected.[35] This transforms the possibility of dialogue, and therefore of consolation. The face-to-face relationship between two people presupposes the possibility of time, of passing between past and future: conversely, this passage is a condition of the intersubjective relationship.[36] The condition of time lies in the relationship between humans or in history. As one waits for death, one is

> cut adrift from one's future, and from one's past. One knows that what is coming is death ... All the experience and skills one has acquired are powerless to deal with it. As the imminence of death looms, it cuts one adrift from one's past. There is nothing to do but suffer and wait for death. One is held in the suffering, in the pain, in the present. The present stretches on, without passing, without going anywhere ...[37]

The moment of transition to palliative care can often be very painful for all concerned. This is because of the existential transformation that is involved, the extinguishment of the future, the immersion in being, the overwhelming presence of the sense of physical being, the aloneness that disconnects from speech. Sometimes dying people reflect painfully on their pasts, sometimes—like the old Count Bolkonsky in *War and Peace*—they try to make amends for their mistakes, sometimes they are merely disappointed that nothing profound or inspiring occurs to them. Whatever the quality of the experience, the conditions for dialogue are profoundly transformed: one talks to a dying person differently from how one talks to a person who is not dying.

******

The moral specificity of palliative care arises out of its distinctive goals and the ways in which it seeks to achieve them. The objectives of palliation and relief of symptoms colour most of the decisions that are made. These decisions can certainly be complex and controversial, especially where there's uncertainty about whether hydration should be provided or sedation should be given, or where the patient asks for help with dying. The relationship structure of palliative care is also distinctive: rather than relying almost entirely on the dyadic relationship of the clinic, care is provided in a team setting, by doctors, nurses, relatives and others.[38] In Maria's case, I was pleased to be allowed to participate.

The team aspect of palliative care is one of its most distinctive features and has more than just strategic value. Classically, medical care is delivered through a one-to-one relationship between doctor and patient that is closely structured but fluid in content, and which deploys present experiences to interrogate the past and to make projections into the future. This model provides a powerful basis for questioning both biological and psychological processes. The emphasis of palliative care, however, is not on radical interrogation but on comfort and alleviation of symptoms, which is more effectively promoted in the setting of a community of carers. Here, the prohibition within the medical relationship against empathy and reciprocity is reversed, and replaced by a deliberate attempt to provide affirmation and support. Of course, the 'community' of the hospice is not a fully authentic community, and it only partially replaces the traditional relationships that gave way to the mass society that arose along with scientific medicine. Nonetheless, artifice or not, it provides an effective setting for supportive care, allows coordination of care and—importantly—provides an explicit place for relatives and friends.

In the classical doctor–patient relationship, family members scarcely figure at all.[39] By contrast, in the network of relationships underlying palliative care, they are recognised not only as important contributors to the caring process but also as in need of care themselves. Sometimes this dual role—and indeed, the team structure itself—raises delicate issues. Should relatives be consulted before the patient herself? Should information—including private and intimate details—be shared among all members of the team? How should differences of opinion be resolved? Who assumes responsibility for difficult decisions?

Naturally, as with all ethical questions, there aren't any general answers. As always, decisions depend on the specific details of the relationships involved and the processes of dialogue that emerge from them. In Maria's case, her husband participated in many of the team discussions. Maria herself remained subdued and taciturn, although she made an effort to rise to the occasion when Elena, now five and obviously suffering herself, came in to visit. I visited frequently, pretending—I don't really know why—that I was attending the hospice to see other patients and that I was just looking in incidentally to see how she was. I was genuinely interested in Maria and felt a compulsion to see her illness through to the end. However, during my visits she gave little away.

After a few days, Maria announced that she had decided to go home. I sensed her feeling that her last days were being taken from her, conventionalised, medicalised, and I thought back to her comment during that rushed conversation about choosing the style of her own death. Going home was a difficult undertaking, since she required constant care, including with respect to bowel and bladder function. Nonetheless, the team supported the decision and elaborate arrangements were quickly made for a trial visit. A couple of days later she left, with Brian and Elena in an optimistic frame of mind.

By now, however, not much could go right. The home visit was a complete disaster. It immediately became clear that despite all the supports there was no way she could stay there for more than a very short period. In panic and despair, her husband called the ambulance to take her back to the hospice. Their return was like a funeral procession.

The next day, Maria announced in what had become her familiar monotone that she had come to the realisation that she would never be able to live a life that satisfied the minimum conditions she demanded and that she was now ready to die. In this, she asked the treating doctors and nurses for help. Her husband, speechless with despair, sat silently by her bed and made no response at all. The members of the team shifted uneasily on their feet. Eventually, someone suggested that they retire to a neighbouring room to talk over what they should do.

******

Although the questions of euthanasia and assisted suicide have attracted a great deal of public attention and debate, there is little support for these practices among palliative carers.[40] Proponents of legalisation of assisted dying argue that society has no right to interfere with the free choice of individuals to decide how they die, that it is just a simple matter of a right to self-determination.[41] They contend that active intervention to end a life is rational and appropriate where there is intractable pain or other distressing symptoms that are unresponsive to treatment. Potential benefits for society are also mentioned, such as savings on scarce health care resources that could be applied for purposes more socially beneficial than needless prolongation of life. It is argued that euthanasia and assisted suicide are in any case widely practised, as has been shown by many surveys of doctors and nurses[42], and that it is surely better to allow the practice to occur openly and subject to clearly defined rules than surreptitiously, without regulation.

Opponents of euthanasia and assisted suicide respond that requests for assistance in dying are, in fact, usually indications of inadequate palliative care, social support systems for the dying, poor attitudes and practices of practitioners, or maybe of the presence of fears of death, pain, dependence or of becoming a burden, or the existence of psychiatric disease. They point to evidence that where palliative care is provided, unrelieved pain occurs in very few cases[43], and that psychiatric morbidity among patients requesting physician-hastened death is considerable.[44] In all these cases, they argue, the correct response is not to kill the patient but to rectify the relevant deficiency, using whatever therapies are available, including psychosocial and pharmacological approaches.[45] Furthermore, they claim, preservation and protection of life are fundamental values of medicine that would be put at risk if doctors were allowed also to be executioners. They also contend that if euthanasia were to become accepted in any form, it would be impossible to prevent either its gradual extension—for example, to non-terminal conditions and non-voluntary euthanasia—or pressure being brought to bear on the elderly to die rather than continuing to live and imposing a burden on their families or the wider society.[46] In addition, they say, the widespread availability of euthanasia would provide an excuse for policymakers to avoid providing adequate resources to care for the elderly, and would devalue ageing and erode trust in medicine generally. In any case, they dispute the existence of a supposed autonomous right to request and receive euthanasia or physician-assisted suicide, either on religious or on philosophical grounds.[47]

The debate is vigorous and continuing, and there are many more arguments on both sides, including those that purport to draw lessons—positive or negative—from the experiences in jurisdictions in which some degree of legalisation has occurred, such as the Netherlands, the American state of Oregon, and the Northern Territory of Australia. At this stage, it is possible to say only that it is clear that no particular point of view prevails, and that maybe no definitive resolution will ever occur. Indeed, it may even be better to leave the matter unresolved as a matter of principle and to promote the ongoing discussion as a healthy social process, though in this case the legal problem would have to be addressed of how to allow individuals within communities to make their own decisions while preserving healthy, moral debate.

In Maria's case, when the team re-emerged the decision was, perhaps not surprisingly, that the request for euthanasia was denied. Although it was accepted that her condition was a terminal one, the doctor told her, the view had prevailed that there was no imminent threat to her life. Apart from the disease in the spinal column, there was no evidence of spread of tumour elsewhere and she seemed to have no other medical conditions. He told Maria that should pain or other distressing symptoms develop, she would be given whatever treatment was needed to control them. Arrangements would also be made for her to be assessed by a psychiatrist and to be visited by a psychologist and an occupational therapist.

******

We do not know what Maria was thinking as the verdict regarding her request for euthanasia was being delivered. According to the people I have spoken to who were there, her face remained impassive and she didn't make a sound. But when the doctor finished and the team was shuffling out the door, she was heard to mutter a muffled 'Goodbye'. As far as I can ascertain, that was the last word she was heard to speak. In retrospect, it is clear that her mind must already have been made up when she made the request. She had decided that for her, the end had come. She'd tried everything—orthodox medicine, alternative medicine, religion, palliative care. Now she had reached the end of the road.

From that moment on—it was a Monday morning—she merely sat, as in a trance, silent and expressionless. She did not respond to the comings and goings in the ward. She did not answer when she was offered food or drink. The evening came and she had not moved. Her husband and daughter visited, sat with her for a bit, and left.

When the morning came, she was dead.

******

More than ten years have passed since Maria's death, but those last hours remain frozen in my memory. I have moved on to other things, as no doubt also have the other people who had contact with her. However, the story stays with me, a constant source of perplexity. Like the Ancient Mariner, I wearily tell it again and again, trying to make sense, trying to understand what decision, what word, might have caused things to turn out differently.

I don't know what happened to Brian and Elena. Elena must be sixteen now—a young woman. I often wonder how she thinks of her mother, and of her struggle and eventual death. I wonder, too, whether it would have been better if Maria had given in more graciously and died as a mere hospital statistic—as she herself put it—rather than as she did, perversely, in anger or despair, spiting us all. Perhaps it would have been easier for us that way. On the other hand, maybe it was she who was right: after all, she did gain two years free from disease and the disciplinary structures of institutional medicine. And she did manage to die in her own way, at a time of her own choosing.

I don't know why I am so troubled by the story and its outcome. Nor do I know what is achieved by constantly going over it. Despite her determination, Maria was defeated in her struggle, as we knew from the start she would be. Perhaps it worries me that there is nothing to show after all the struggle and all the pain. Nothing, that is, except perhaps the faint traces left in the lives of those she touched and the fact that I, at least, remain to bear witness to the story.

Notes

1. For example, F Randall and DS Downie, *Palliative Care Ethics: A Companion for All Specialities* (Oxford, Oxford University Press, 1998).
2. See Chapter 2.
3. S Kierkegaard, *The Sickness unto Death* (New York, Doubleday Anchor, 1954), p. 158.
4. F Dostoyevsky, *The Idiot* (Middlesex, Penguin, 1955), pp. 90–3.
5. M Merleau-Ponty, *The Visible and the Invisible* (Evanston, North-western University Press, 1968).

6. E Levinas, *Time and the Other* (Pittsburgh, PA, Duquesne University Press, 1987), p. 67.
7. M Heidegger, *The Concept of Time* (Oxford, Blackwell, 1989), p. 7E.
8. ibid., pp. 13E–14E.
9. ibid., p. 20E. cf. M Heidegger, *Being and Time* (Oxford, Blackwell, 1978), pp. 279–312.
10. M Heidegger, *The Concept of Time*, p. 21E.
11. ibid., p. 11E.
12. H Arendt, *Eichmann in Jerusalem: A Report on the Banality of Evil* (Harmondsworth, Penguin, 1977), p. 106.
13. E Scarry, *The Body in Pain: The Making and Unmaking of the World* (Oxford, Oxford University Press, 1985), p. 57.
14. A Lingis, *Dangerous Emotions* (Berkeley, University of California Press, 2000).
15. G Agamben, *Remnants of Auschwitz: The Witness and the Archive* (New York, Zone Books, 1999).
16. E Bloch, *The Principle of Hope* (Boston, MA, MIT Press, 1995).
17. E Ernst and BR Cassileth, 'The Prevalence of Complementary/Alternative Medicine in Cancer', *Cancer*, 83, 1998: 777–82.
18. This paragraph and the next rely heavily on the argument in I Illich, *Limits to Medicine. Medical Nemesis: The Appropriation of Health* (London, Marion Boyars, 1976), chapters 2, 5.
19. See N Barley, *Dancing on the Grave: Encounters with Death* (London, Abacus, 1995); R Peile, *Body and Soul: An Aboriginal View* (Carlisle, Western Australia, Hesperion Press, 1997), chapter 1.
20. I Illich, *Limits to Medicine*, p. 103, n. 209.
21. cf. M Weber, 'Science as a Vocation', in H Gerth and CW Mills, eds, *From Max Weber* (New York, Routledge, 1998).
22. I Illich, *Limits to Medicine*, p. 190.
23. See also D Callaghan, *The Troubled Dream of Life: Living with Mortality* (New York, Simon and Schuster, 1993), chapter 1.
24. I Illich, *Limits to Medicine*, p. 200.
25. E Cassell, 'Dying in a Technical Society', *Hastings Centre Report*, 2, May 1974: 31–6.
26. I Illich, *Limits to Medicine*, p. 107–8.
27. P Ariès, *The Hour of Our Death* (New York, Alfred A. Knopf, 1981).
28. See, for example, WB Forman, *Hospice and Palliative Care: Concepts and Practice* (Boston, Jones & Bartlett, 2003).
29. MA Ashby and B Stoffell, 'Therapeutic Ration and Defined Phases: Proposal of an Ethical Framework for Palliative Care', *Brit Med J*, 302, 1991: 1322–4.
30. cf. T Horwitz, 'My Death', in J Malpas and RC Solomon, eds, *Death and Philosophy* (London, Routledge, 1998), pp. 5–16; M Heidegger, *Being and Time*, pp. 281–5.
31. A Lingis, *Dangerous Emotions*.
32. E Levinas, *Totality and Infinity* (Pittsburgh, Duquesne University Press, 1969), p. 238.

33 E Levinas, *Time and the Other*, pp. 70–1.
34 E Levinas, *Totality and Infinity*, pp. 232–5.
35 A Lingis, *Dangerous Emotions*.
36 E Levinas, *Time and the Other*, p. 79.
37 A Lingis, *Dangerous Emotions*. For a discussion about the experience of serious illness, see also A Frank, *At the Will of the Body: Reflections on Illness* (Boston, Houghton Mifflin Co., 1991).
38 F Randall and DS Downie, *Palliative Care Ethics*, chapter 4.
39 cf. R Zaner, *Ethics and the Clinical Encounter* (Englewood Cliffs, NJ, Prentice Hall, 1988), chapter 3.
40 R Woodruff, 'Euthanasia and Physician-Assisted Suicide—Are They Clinically Necessary?', International Hospice Institute and College, http://hospicecare.com.
41 See, for example, J Rachels, *The End of Life* (New York, Oxford University Press, 1986); D Callaghan, *The Troubled Dream of Life: In Search of a Peaceful Death* (New York, Touchstone, 1993); H Kuhse, *The Sanctity of Life Doctrine in Medicine* (Oxford, Clarendon Press, 1987).
42 F Starace and L Sherr, 'Suicidal Behaviours, Euthanasia and AIDS', *AIDS*, 12, 1998: 339–47; DE Meier, CA Emons, S Wallenstein et al., 'A National Survey of Physician-assisted Suicide and Euthanasia in the United States', *N Engl J Med*, 338, 1998: 1193–201.
43 NI Cherny and R Catane, 'Professional Negligence in the Management of Cancer Pain: A Case for Urgent Reforms', *Cancer*, 76, 1995: 2181–5.
44 HM Chochinov and KG Wilson, 'The Euthanasia Debate: Attitudes, Practices and Psychiatric Considerations', *Can J Psych*, 40, 1995: 593–602; W Breitbart and BD Rosenfeld, 'Physician-assisted Suicide: The Influence of Psychosocial Issues', *Cancer Control*, 6, 1999: 146–61.
45 RM Cole, 'Communicating with People who Request Euthanasia', *Palliat Med*, 7, 1993: 139–43.
46 RG Twycross, 'Euthanasia: Going Dutch?', *J R Soc Med*, 89, 1996: 61–3.
47 PA Singer and M Siegler, 'Euthanasia—A Critique', *N Engl J Med*, 322, 1990: 1881–3.

CHAPTER 9

Time, Ethics and the Archive

> I have heard the mermaids singing, each to each.
> I do not think that they will sing to me.
> I have seen them riding seaward on the waves
> combing the white hair of the waves blown back
> when the wind blows the water white and black.
> We have lingered in the chambers of the sea
> By sea-girths wreathed with seaweed red and brown
> Till human voices wake us, and we drown.[1]

Elizabeth was three years old when she and her mother left home. She can remember it all vividly. It was a hot, stifling summer's night. The plan had been carefully worked out. She pretended to be asleep, while in reality she was lying under the covers fully dressed. She was nervous, trembling. She was wearing her red shoes and the dress with the little roses on it, and she had her favourite spotty ribbon in her hair. The light from the streetlight outside the window cast long shadows across the room. She didn't know why they were going on such a strange adventure so late at night. When the house was quiet her mother came in and signalled to her. Silently, they left the house and crept to the railway station where they caught a train. It was hot and late and she was aching with tiredness. They made their way to the house of a friend of her mother and slept on the floor. Over the next few weeks they moved house many times. Eventually they set up in another city.

Elizabeth had been close to her father and had loved him very much. He had played with her and indulged her, often bringing her presents. The ribbon had been one of these presents. She had had no inkling of trouble between her parents and to this day does not understand why her mother left. She never saw her father again.

******

A moment in time can alter one's entire life. It can change everything. It can transform one's experience of oneself and of other people. A single event can interrupt the flow of a life and set it on a new course.

We depend on the continuity of our internal time to maintain the integrity of our face-to-face engagements with others—indeed, to constitute both ourselves and these relationships. We confront each other in time, with a view to a common future. The present is the crystallisation of complex pasts. The future is generated out of the past in the flux of these face-to-face encounters.

The present—now, here, for me—is not only a modality of time: it is also an inherent component of social being. It signifies the presence of another for me. When the threads that tie the past to the future are broken, a fissure propagates through all the layers of our experience.

******

Elizabeth took the loss of her father very hard. She would try to remember what he looked like, and to imagine that he was with her, playing their favourite games. She slept with the ribbon under her pillow. Then, for years, she was angry with him for not having tried to find her. Eventually, she discovered the truth—he had written many letters to her mother pleading to be able to see his daughter, but, having received no reply, in the end returned in despair to his native Italy. By the time she herself wrote, it was too late: the message came back that, tragically, he had died the previous year.

******

The time of memory is not the same as clock time. Nor are the meanings of memories the same as those of the linear narratives within which they were once embedded. Memories inhabit a symbolic domain that has both a logic and a dynamic of its own. This is not to say that one can generalise without restraint about the meanings of memories—or, for that matter, of dreams. The contents of particular symbols can only be fixed in relation to the specific details of an individual's fund of experiences, in relation, so to speak, to the texture of a particular lifeworld.

But on the other hand, the experience of time is not a purely individual phenomenon. Time is a constitutive variable of all social life and a common condition of the identities of those who confront each other in social encounters. Further, time and memory are represented either in speech or in writing, either in private reflection or in public discourse, through complex plays of signification embedded in language. Narratives of personal experience, therefore—of lives, of illnesses—have temporal structures that fix ethical values and meanings.

In Elizabeth's case, no-one can presume from general considerations to understand the meaning of the memories of that night, of the flight from her home, of the shadows, the dress, the shoes, the ribbon. These can only be explicated in the concrete, in the particular.

> The remembered *is past*, a strange intensity of not now and most surely now. An intension of time … not … of agency, an intensity of loss and beginning, an intensity that moves people, affects them, gives them to see things in particular ways. The remembered is not only not now but is at once now and possibly yet to be …[2]

******

Fifty-five years have gone by since the day they left. Many things have happened, but Elizabeth has not been able to escape—the room, the flower dress, the red shoes, the loss. She can't smell the hot air of a summer night without evoking the tragic rupture in her life. She still has the ribbon, which she takes out from time to time to look at and to feel against her cheek.

In the time I have known Elizabeth—it must be nearly a decade now—she has told the story maybe a dozen times. She wants to understand, she says, but cannot do so. She wants to understand why it happened, and why she has never known what happiness is.

******

A large part of the work of a doctor involves the organisation of memories, listening to reminiscences, piecing together stories, constructing histories. Each of these activities involves the mobilisation of a particular discursive system and a particular modality of time. The use of a scientific narrative invokes the linear temporality—the so-called 'objective time' of biology and physics. Other modalities of time play an important role in medicine, in shaping meanings and values. Sense only arises in relation to defined discursive systems, and medicine subserves several such systems, including the articulation of private experiences, the construction of a narrative of illness and health, and psychological and social discourses.

The doctor's task is both to interpret the narratives of the patient and to construct new ones. He or she stands as a witness to the sufferings of the patient, as does the patient herself, although in a rather different manner. As described earlier, there are two meanings of the word 'witness': there is 'the survivor', the person who has lived through an experience, and there is the person who observes from the outside, as in a lawsuit between two parties.[3] In the setting of medicine, the former describes the position of the patient who has lived through an illness from beginning to end and has acquired knowledge about it from the inside, while the latter describes that of the doctor, as one who observes, who sees from the outside, who records the suffering. In his role as a witness, the doctor is a repository of stored meanings, the creator and keeper of an active memory, an archive, so to speak, that records and organises the experiences of the patient (a witness in the other sense), thereby rendering them intelligible and therefore bearable. By constructing such an archive[4], the doctor becomes a custodian of the past, a timekeeper, who defines the telos of past events and points to future possibilities.

> I have seen the moment of my greatness flicker,
> And I have seen the eternal Footman hold my coat and
>   snicker,
> And, in short, I was afraid.[5]

Elizabeth loved sport. She was a keen sportswoman—not a champion, but a good performer. She ran, played basketball, and swam. Never very good at school, she was nonetheless respected for her physical prowess. She prized her health and vigour and was proud of her stamina. Looking back, she says now that this was the only time in her life she knew a sense of promise, of hope and open possibilities. In fact, she has a photograph of herself from this time that she carries around with her, which she will show with a little prompting. I have never asked about the circumstances in which it was taken. It shows a slim, dark-haired woman, attractive but not beautiful, perhaps a little sad, perhaps with a faint smile, looking defiantly, into the camera.

Elizabeth always found it difficult to develop intimate friendships. After a few disastrous love affairs with married men, she settled on a marriage with Tom, a factory worker fifteen years older than herself. It was not much of a relationship from the start, as she will readily confess. He drank too hard and couldn't find regular work. He had a job in the car industry for a few years, but when that ended and the recession hit, things got bad. They had a daughter, Dee, to whom she was completely devoted.

Around age thirty she started to experience odd sensations in her arms and legs, as well as dizziness and occasional blurring of vision. At first she ignored these feelings. Maybe she was just dong too much running or swimming. She cut down a bit, watched her diet. Things settled down. A year or so later, the symptoms returned. Tom was drinking again and became violent when she complained. They never had any money.

Her symptoms became worse. She went to doctors. They tried to reassure her. Depression. Anxiety. More doctors. Chronic fatigue. Just rest, they said. But she was scared now. She felt something was wrong. She couldn't run or swim any more. Her body was betraying her. She would recall the happy little girl in the flower dress, the pristine purity of the room, of the mythic time of certainty and love. She had experienced her moment of promise, the time when her future was open, when she had heard the mermaids singing. It hadn't lasted long.

******

For Elizabeth, time was out of joint, just as it had been for the young Hamlet. She confronted a discontinuity, an interruption—not for the first time in her life. Lived time, the time of the body and of lived experience, with its rhythms and its cadences, follows a different logic to physical time. Now this time, these rhythms, were—once again—discordant, cacophonous.

As Deleuze explains, the joints, or hinges, of time are the transition points through which the periodic movements it measures pass. In ancient philosophy, time was subordinated to the circular movement of the world. It was like a labyrinth opening onto an eternal origin[6], and entailed 'an entire hierachization of movements according to … their necessity, their perfection, their uniformity, their rotation, their composite spirals, and the numbers of time that correspond to them'.[7]

As long as time stays on its hinges, it remains the measure of movement, its interval or number. When time is out of joint, however, it is no longer related to the movement it measures. Rather, movement becomes dependent on the time that conditions it. Moreover, 'movement is no longer the determination of objects, but the description of a space, a space we must set aside in order to discover time as the condition of action. Time thus becomes unilinear and rectilinear …'[8]

The fateful predicament recognised by Hamlet—the tension between a complex, organic, lived time and an external, linear abstract one—has been a condition of life since the age of Enlightenment. The time of science—'objective' time—continually threatens to overwhelm, to supplant, the multiplicity of other modalities of time embedded in social and personal life. The pure order of time is now taken to define the parts of movements, inasmuch as they are determined within it. The experiences of permanence, succession and simultaneity become no more than abstract modes or relations of time. The 'labyrinth' of time takes on a new look—neither a circle nor a spiral, but now a single thread, pure and straight, all the more mysterious in that it is simple, inexorable, terrible: in the words of Borges.[9]

The opposition of linear time to the topologically complex cadences of immanent time, of the arrow of infinite progression to the whirligig of eternal return, is nowhere more intense than in the experience of illness and its representation within medicine. The linear time of science provides a potent tool for the analysis of pathological disturbances in the functioning of tissues, but it always remains external to the phenomena it is applied to to explain. For the sufferer herself, however, it provides no possibility of solace, because in the event of failure it leaves no way out, apart from the abyss of the future.

******

In his phenomenological analysis of time, Husserl shows how time and temporal objects are constituted.[10] He demonstrates how, in my field of presence, I make contact with time and learn to know its course.[11] In his famous analysis of the network of intentionalities in temporal perception, he shows how the 'protentions', or anticipations, and 'retentions', or perceptual memories, combine to constitute the living present as duration, and how these intentionalities do not run from a central I but from my perceptual field itself, which draws along in its wake its own horizon of retentions and with its protentions bites into the future.[12]

In this way, Husserl shows how the living present in fact has both depth and continuity, making the presence of objects possible. He demonstrates how this thick 'now' is grasped in a quasi-immediacy that does not require, and must be radically distinguished from, separate acts of remembering that would attempt to repeat and reproduce the occurrence.[13]

While Husserl's account focuses on time consciousness itself, other thinkers, such as Heidegger and Levinas, have shown how this experience lies at the basis of both individual identity and social experience. According to them, temporality is one of the fundamental conditions by which we recognise ourselves as individuals, either alone or in relation to others.[14] The passage between past and future is also a condition of intersubjective relationships, or rather, the intertwining of beings that are immanently social[15], and, in particular, of the face-to-face relationship between people. Therefore, time lies at the heart of the ethical bond, which only exists in time, as a flux of relationships with both a future and a past.[16]

The experiences associated with illness interrupt the flux of lived time and thereby challenge the continuity of the ethical bond. Illness problematises the future and raises questions about the meaning of the past. Sometimes this can be a fruitful and creative process; at other times, it can be destructive or even dangerous. The pathologies of time associated with illness can be very complex. The awareness of mortality, the fear of serious disability, sometimes even minor illnesses, can generate transformed, abrogated relationships with both the future and the past.[17] The intentional threads can be loosened, or broken altogether.

******

With an increasing sense of foreboding, Elizabeth went from doctor to doctor. Eventually, one came up with a possible diagnosis. It could be multiple sclerosis, he muttered matter of factly, half to himself. She remembers the moment well, as vividly as the flower dress night. Although at the time she had no idea what the term signified, his words struck her with the force of a hammer. Her head reeled, her eyes clouded, the sounds of the outside world became dim. The doctor continued to talk on in a monotone, but she heard no more words. She can't remember the rest of the consultation—thanking him, saying goodbye, perhaps paying the bill. She staggered out into the street. Everything was spinning. She didn't know where she was or what she should do.

******

We are all familiar with moments where time stands still, where the intensity of an experience seems to overwhelm the inexorable flux of temporal succession. The instant before impact in a motor car accident; the moment one is confronted by an assailant in the street, or hears of the death of a world leader; the moment of climax in a theatre performance, or a football game. Perhaps when one receives a death sentence, either literally or figuratively.[18] Such nodal points shape the temporal landscape, draw together the expanse of memory into a series of punctuations, stops and renewals.

Every moment, in fact, has a depth or intensity of its own[19], which redirects attention away from the dull homogeneity of succession to the sharpness of discrete experiences. In general, time is thought of, memory is constructed, from within the ecstasy of eternal moments.[20] In his book *Twilight of the Idols*, Nietzsche drew particular attention to this 'intoxication' or 'rapture' of the moment, the feeling of plenitude and increased energy[21], in which one 'enriches everything out of one's own abundance'. 'What one sees', Nietzsche says, 'what one desires, one sees swollen, pressing, strong, overladen with energy'.[22] At the particular moments of profound intensity, at the nodal points, this experience is heightened still further. It as if 'time [has] flown away', as if I have 'fallen … into [what he called] the well of eternity'.[23]

The experience of the intensity of the moment can be either positive or negative. The moment anticipated, and later encountered, by Faust was one of ecstatic liberation and exaltation. Elizabeth too had fallen into a well of eternity. But for her, the moment was not one of unbounded happiness but of uncertainty and, ultimately, despair.

> For I have known them all already, known them all—
> Have known the evenings, mornings, afternoons,
> I have measured out my life with coffee spoons;
> I know the voices dying with a dying fall
> Beneath the music from a farther room.[24]

Ten years later, Elizabeth is sitting in my office. She can now barely walk. Tom has emphysema and heart failure, but still drinks and is more abusive than ever. He'll never work again. Things have not gone well for them. They live off their combined pensions, which give them so little money that they can scarcely afford to eat.

We talk. She tells me about her medical problems, in relation to which I provide assistance. She's had a lot of them: bladder and bowel dysfunction, broken bones, a stroke. Her eyesight has been affected and her speech is beginning to deteriorate. The course appears now to be one of inexorable decline. She doesn't complain. She has never complained. She displays complete equanimity: What can you do? she asks. I wonder if such passivity comes out of all her personal tragedies, whether they have so numbed her that she cannot respond to injustice, cannot hope any more.

As usual, the conversation turns to her father. Today, she is wondering if she inherited her medical conditions from him. Her mother, whom she rarely sees, is nearly eighty and well. Then she talks about

Dee, who is a young woman now. She is a promising basketball player but probably won't make professional grade.

I accompany Elizabeth outside as we are finishing and meet Dee, who has come to pick her up. I am jolted by the resemblance to the girl in the photo. She has the same blush of youth, the same sad smile. There is a sense of the uncanny about it: for a moment I am staring straight back through the years, to the time before the start of Elizabeth's decline, to that fleeting moment of promise that was never realised.

******

Although in medicine we talk of the 'natural history' of an illness, in reality no such thing exists. The course of every illness is unique, varying in relation to the specific physiological, psychological and social contexts of the individuals who experience them. These contexts are themselves historically conditioned. Changes in the patterns of work and leisure, of diet and the quality of the environment, the development of new drugs or other forms of treatment, all become part of this so-called evolving 'natural' history. Similarly, the meanings of an illness are constructed in relation to shared social traditions and cultural valuations.

In other words, disease and illness are complex constructions that bring together a range of semiotic variables, discursive systems and narrative realisations. Accordingly, they are subject to variation in several intersecting dimensions, including the dimensions of causation, of biological effects on tissues, of therapeutic approaches and techniques, of formal description and organisation of disease phenomena, of social meanings and ethical values, and of individual personal experiences of illness. Thus, Elizabeth's story comprises her personal narrative and mine, the various cultural constructions associated with her diagnosis and her disability, and the implications for, and effects on, her friends and family and the wider society.

The recognition of the complex semiotic content of illness and narrative, of the various modalities of illness stories, however, raises the question of the nature of their relationship to time. Indeed, semiological analysis has tended to depreciate the role of temporal variables within such multilayered assemblies. Roland Barthes put it this way:

All contemporary researchers ... could subscribe to [the] ... proposition that the order of chronological succession is absorbed in an atemporal structure. [For them,] Temporality is only a structural category of (discourse); from the point of view of narrative, what we call time does not exist, or at least only as an element of a semiotic system.[25]

But how can a sign incorporate a temporal dimension, and what is the relationship between the present instant as experienced by an individual, no matter how 'thick' or laden with meaning, and the broad historical context of the society in which he or she lives? At the level of her personal life, within her own lifeworld, how does Elizabeth experience the passage of time? Husserl's phenomenological analysis showed how the experience of the living present depended on the self-identity of the now as a point as it appears in a field of presence, which maintains links with the flux of retentions and protentions. In fact—as Jacques Derrida has shown—the signs on which we depend to shape and to render meaningful even our most rudimentary perceptions, inherently involve temporal determinations. Signification and hence language are immanently temporal.[26] Meanings are generated by the play of signs only out of the differences between them, only out of, so to speak, the shifting spaces revealed by the process of signification. This process of deferral is built into the terms, and thus constitutes an inherent dynamic process. Signs are 'traces' that involve a similar relation to an imaginary time, an imaginary relation to an origin. Textual constructions, narratives, are 'movements of an impossible desire for plenitude, presence'.

The experience of being in time, then, possesses its own specific features that are not reducible to those of a linear time, of a neutral series of abstract moments. The time of the simplest narrative escapes the ordinary notion of time, conceived of as a series of instants succeeding one another along an abstract line oriented in a single direction.[27] The time of the narrative, furthermore, is public time, in that it engages the dynamic of semiotic systems and the cultural investments of signs. The fibres of one's experience of an illness, either as a sufferer or as an observer, are bound together by temporal threads. The simplest form of expressivity—the description of a symptom, a cry of pain—is inherently temporal, in the sense that it could not exist without time, and at the same time brings time into existence.

The narrative text is a powerful force for the transformation of time. The nature of this transformation, however, is rather different from that confronted with such poignancy by Hamlet: indeed, the movement here is in precisely the opposite direction. The text frees interpretation from the constraints of linearity and generates a more complex, multidimensional experience of meaning. Memory need no longer be seen as a personal narrative of external adventures stretching along episodic time. It can be recognised as possessing a more complex structure, as a spiral movement that, through anecdotes and episodes, brings us back to the almost motionless constellation of potentialities that the narrative retrieves. In this sense, narrative functions to provide a transition from internal time consciousness to historicality.[28]

******

Tom died last year. Elizabeth was philosophical. It hadn't been a good relationship. He was cruel to her, beat her, didn't provide much. But he was her husband. She had made a choice and accepted responsibility for it. She looked after him to the end. My impression is that she gave more to him that he gave to her, but you really never know. They had eked out an honourable life together, as indigent and suffused with pain as it was. The indigence did not end with his death either. With Tom gone, Elizabeth's pension was cut by half. She couldn't afford many of her drugs anymore and had to stop several of them. She has ended up in hospital a few times as a result.

Elizabeth is not bitter. Not about the night in the floral dress. Not about her fatherless childhood and adolescence. Not about her thwarted hopes and unrealised ambitions. Not about her illness, pain and disability. Not even about Tom.

She still has the spotty ribbon. It is her most prized possession. It symbolises for her all the things she never had: the security of unconditional love, protection against the harshness and cruelty of daily existence, hope and confidence that the future might be different.

******

In the world of texts, discourses and narratives of personal experience, there is no one time. Rather, there are multiple times, or multiple dimensions along which temporality might be plotted. There is the time of language, of society and culture, of science; there is psychological time, emotional time, the time of suffering and of loving. The various texts that go to make up a story fit together in unpredictable and fluid ways: within them, time can be pluralised and expanded, or contracted and interrupted.

The archive that is constructed through the clinical dialogue is not an undifferentiated mass of statements that 'unifies everything that has been said in the great, confused murmur of a discourse'. Rather, it is a dynamic, reflective system that governs the appearance of statements as unique events, which 'differentiates discourses in their multiple existence and specifies them in their own duration'[29]; that is, the clinical archive recognises the multiple voices, themes and strata of the clinic and seeks to accommodate them within a topographic schema that allows them to preserve their distinctive character but nevertheless engage each other in a kind of internal dialogue.

The spiral trajectories of signification and narrative in relation to the various dimensions of time undermine the possibility of fixed identities at the root of social interchanges, and, therefore, of monolithic value systems arising in relation to these multiple modes of social life. These cycles of change, of completed wholeness, thus convey ethical outcomes. They ensure that ethical decisions are understood in terms of their infinite implications, in relation to their complex roles at all levels of personal and social meaning.

The archaeology of time also draws our attention to the dialectical relationship between the universal, or global, and the singular, or local, within ethics in medicine. Despite all the attempts at universal formulations, ethical discourses are subject to both irreducible singularity and infinite complexity. The ethical content of an interaction is constituted not by universal principles, nor by local contextual features seen as empirical facts or conditions. It is constituted by multiple dimensions of actions and interactions, by the fact and character of its localness.

******

Elizabeth's life goes on. She has seen the moment of her greatness flicker. She has known the dying voices in the farther room. She has heard the mermaids singing, even if they did not sing for her.

But her time is not yet over. A great expanse has been traversed between the woman, prematurely aged, beset by pain and disability, violence and poverty, and the little girl in the stifling room half a century before.

A great expanse in one sense, but in another nothing at all. In her journey through the dark, incessant labyrinth, she has hardly left her point of origin. All the key events, the hopes and the disappointments, are still there, here, now, bound together by that ribbon of memories, stories and narratives in the great, continuing archive of her life.

Notes

1. TS Eliot, 'The Love Song of J. Alfred Prufrock', in *Selected Poems* (UK, Faber and Faber, 1954).
2. CE Scott, *The Time of Memory* (Albany, NY, SUNY Press, 1999), p. 54.
3. See Chapter 6 and G Agamben, *Remnants of Auschwitz: The Witness and the Archive* (New York, Zone Books, 1999), p. 17.
4. ibid.
5. TS Eliot, 'The Love Song of J. Alfred Prufrock'.
6. G Deleuze, 'On Four Poetic Formulas that Might Summarise the Kantian Philosophy', in G Deleuze, *Essays, Critical and Clinical*, tr. DW Smith and MA Greco (Minneapolis, University of Minnesota Press, 1997), pp. 27–35.
7. ibid., p. 27.
8. ibid., pp. 27–9.
9. JL Borges, 'Death and the Compass', in *Ficciones*, tr. A Kerrigan (New York, Knopf, 1993), p. 113, quoted by G Deleuze, *Essays, Critical and Clinical*.
10. E Husserl, *The Phenomenology of Internal Time Consciousness* (Bloomington, Indiana University Press, 1973).
11. M Merleau-Ponty, The Phenomenology of Perception (London, Routledge and Kegan Paul, 1960), p. 416.
12. ibid.
13. ibid.
14. M Heidegger, *The Concept of Time* (Oxford, Blackwell, 1989), p. 7E.
15. E Levinas, *Time and the Other* (Pittsburgh, PA, Duquesne University Press, 1987), p. 79.
16. ibid., p. 67.
17. E Levinas, *Totality and Infinity* (Pittsburgh, PA, Duquesne University Press, 1969), pp. 232–5.
18. M Blanchot, *The Instant of My Death*, tr. E Rottenberg (Stanford, CA, Stanford University Press, 2000), pp. 1–11.

19 D Wood, *The Deconstruction of Time* (Evanston, North-western University Press, 1979), p. 20.
20 ibid., p. 21.
21 F Nietzsche, *Twilight of the Idols*, tr. RJ Hollingdale (Middlesex, Penguin, 1974), p. 71.
22 ibid., p. 72. See also M Heidegger, 'The Will to Power as Art', in *Nietzsche*, Volume 1, tr. DF Krell (San Francisco, Harper & Row, 1987).
23 F Nietzsche, *Thus Spake Zarathustra* (New York, Modern Library, 1937), p. 288.
24 TS Eliot, 'The Love Song of J. Alfred Prufrock'.
25 R Barthes, 'Introduction to the Structural Analysis of Narrative', in S Heath, ed., *Image-music-text* (London, Fontana, 1977). cf. D Wood, *The Deconstruction of Time*, p. 348.
26 D Wood, *The Deconstruction of Time*, pp. 330–1.
27 P Ricoeur, 'Narrative Time', *Social Research*, 7; 1980: 169–90.
28 ibid., p. 178.
29 M Foucault, *The Archaeology of Knowledge* (London, Tavistock Publications, 1972), p. 129.

Chapter 10

At the Gates of the Labyrinth
A Meditation on Suffering

> The tide has turned at length:
> Ebb with the tide, drift helpless down,
> Useless to struggle on ...
> How must I deal with grief? ...
> See where my outcast limbs have lain!
> Stones for a bed bring sorrow small relief.
> My heart would burst ...
> For those whom Fate has cursed
> Music itself sings but one note—unending miseries,
>   torment and wrong![1]

I should like to introduce three people I have met over the last year:

Anka was fifteen years old in July 1995. On the day the troops came to Srebrenica, all the people were gathered together in the town centre. Anka's father was the rock of her life, her protector and mentor, a source of knowledge, strength and unlimited love. At first the children thought it was a holiday and were happy, but Anka sensed her father's anxiety. 'Don't worry, my little princess', he said, but she knew he didn't mean it. She watched him standing tensely as she and her mother were bundled into buses and driven away. She never saw him again. Suffering unspeakable privations, the two of them made their way to Germany and eventually to Australia. Now, ten years later, she has learnt her third language, has two university degrees and has just married. She has thought about her father, and her loss, every day. She wonders what he would have thought, whether he would have been proud of what his little princess has been able to accomplish. She continues to draw a deep, sad inspiration from his love. Her sense of loss, however, and her deep wounds, are unabated.

Pimbao Narang lives in a village in northern Thailand with her two children. In 1993 her husband became ill. At first he told her that the doctors had diagnosed cancer but as he neared death, he confessed that he really had AIDS, which he had caught from another woman. By this time Pimbao herself was infected. When she heard the news she was speechless with shock for days. Her first reaction was furious anger but she was able to overcome this and she continued to nurse her husband until he died in her arms. She has since devoted herself to organising a self-help group for women in her village infected with HIV. They come together and make clothes, soft toys and small bags for sale, giving them an income and providing a chance to share their suffering and support each other. She works tirelessly, without any trace of bitterness, despite the debility arising from her own medical condition.

Dr Managayam is the medical superintendent of a hospital on the east coast of Sri Lanka. After the 2004 tsunami struck, he rendered all possible assistance. When I visited him as part of an aid team, he talked to our delegation and listed the needs of his hospital. As we stood to leave, he grabbed my arm and said: 'I must show you the photos'. He took us to his computer and proceeded to show photographs of all 452 people who had died in his village that day. They include children and babies, young men and women, and elderly people. Many were disfigured or horribly bloated from the effects of the water. He went through every photo, frequently exclaiming, 'Look, she is only a baby! *He* is an old man …' When he had finished displaying his grisly inventory, he repeated softly: 'I didn't leave my post. I didn't leave my post …'

******

What is the experience of suffering? How do we make sense of it? Why are we so fascinated by the suffering of others? What effect does it have on us to witness someone in its midst? Is there anything we can learn from it?

I want to tell a story that arose not out of a natural or social catastrophe but, at least on the surface, out of much less spectacular circumstances: the last illness of an old woman. It is a story in which I personally became swept up, and I observed the facts myself or they were related to me by the various protagonists.

******

This is the story of Kakima Oqil and her children. Mrs Oqil was an 85-year-old woman who was dying with bowel cancer after a long, difficult illness. She has three surviving children: her daughter, Sebati, aged fifty-five, and her sons Askhar, aged fifty-nine, and Chajim, aged fifty-seven.

Mrs Oqil had developed abdominal pains two years ago, which caused great distress. For some reason the cause of the pain took many months to diagnose, during which repeated—and, as it turned out, incorrect—reassurances were given that there was no serious underlying problem. During this time, her physical suffering was considerable. She had been admitted to hospital on several occasions with severe, unrelenting pain, but attempts to control it were ineffective. When the diagnosis of metastatic cancer was finally made, the family felt deceived and betrayed. Their trust in their medical advisers was never restored.

Kakima and her husband came from the same small village in Central Europe. They married young and emigrated to Australia in their early twenties. The children were born soon after and the father supported them by working in an engineering factory. Tragically, however, he died in an industrial accident when Sebati was barely two. This was a devastating event for everyone, including Kakima, who had had little education and to that time had never worked in paid employment. Up to her dying days, she would recount the wave of blackness that overcame her when she received the news of her husband's death. With great effort she made a deliberate, conscious decision. This was the great turning point of her life: in one moment she was transformed, from a young wife with a happy family who barely left her house to a determined, tough woman who went forth to do battle with the world.

Out of sheer necessity, and with an obdurate determination for which she became notorious, Kakima stepped into the role of family leader. Her uncompromising toughness surprised even herself. She learned English. She started a small importing business that she steered to success against ruthless competitors. With little education of her own, she supervised the education of her children. As far as can be determined, the possibility of another relationship with a man was never considered.

In her culture, it was the men who usually made the decisions. In the absence of a man, Kakima assumed the role flawlessly and demanded full equality. This and her uncompromising single-mindedness aroused consternation and some antipathy in her community, but she was strong enough to bear that burden and eventually her role and status were grudgingly accepted.

At home, a rigorous regime was enforced. There was little time for recreation. All the children had assigned tasks and punishment was expected if they were not completed. Among themselves, the family spoke the language of Kakima's birth. They were devout Moslems. Kakima selected the future careers of her children: Chajim was to take over the business, Sebati was to obtain a university degree and occupy a professional role, and Askhar was to be the family's support person.

Although she was urged to do so, Sebati never married. Askhar, by contrast, was prohibited from marrying. His task was to care for his siblings, his nieces and nephews and his mother. His contribution was acknowledged—and explicitly referred to within the family—as a 'sacrifice' because it meant not having either children or an education. He worked in factories and at menial jobs to help put his sister and brother through school and university. When his brother's marriage broke up, he looked after the children during the day so that his brother could still go to work. When his mother became ill, he was the one who assumed primary responsibility for her daily care.

Of the three of them, Sebati undoubtedly dominated. She had a strong personality herself and was forceful, well read and articulate. Unlike Askhar's phlegmatic nature, hers was mercurial, temperamental. Like other people of her culture, she tended sometimes to display her feelings with disarming openness. She considered herself blunt but honest. Others no doubt from time to time interpreted her brusque and insistent manner as rude and aggressive.

Sebati was the spokesperson and openly expressed the children's disquietude following her mother's painful illness and the trauma associated with her diagnosis. Perhaps emulating Kakima's own style, she frequently confronted the doctors about decisions they had made, disagreeing with them and questioning closely their judgement and intentions.

******

The experiences of grief and pain are very personal and vary widely. They enter one's familiar, taken-for-granted body and create an infested space within it, reorganising lived space and time, relations with others and with oneself.[2] They produce a state of passivity, helplessness, abandonment and solitude. The comfort and safety of the home, of the familiar dwelling place of the body, are replaced by a sense of transience and contingency.[3] In the setting of illness and hospitalisation, the security of home gives way to the vulnerability incurred by entrusting oneself to the care of a stranger.

Pain and grief are among our most private, isolating experiences. They sap our freedom and ability to act. Pain in particular requires that we give up our freedom, become patients, hand our bodies over to others to probe, palpate, investigate and dissect. At the same time, however, they insinuate a half-opening, 'a half opening that a moan, a cry, a groan or a sigh slips through', an open, fragile call for aid, for help from the other whose alterity promises salvation.[4]

******

Kakima had suffered great pain during her illness. This caused distress and humiliation both to her and to her children. She had experienced pain before, of course: in her culture, the experience of childbirth was never diminished by anaesthetics. But the pain of her illness and the apparent aloof indifference of the medical practitioners had left an indelible impression on the whole family.

Sebati told me one story about this early phase of her mother's illness. On one occasion—when Kakima had been admitted to hospital for investigation—Sebati came to visit and found Kakima crawling on the floor, begging for relief, with doctors and nurses walking by, ignoring her. Sebati called her brothers and they advised the doctors that if this happened again there would be dangerous consequences. Kakima was rapidly discharged from this hospital and did not return.

Kakima herself spoke to me of her pain. In spite of the fact that she had thought that she knew pain well, she had been surprised by how hard it was to bear and was herself deeply resentful of the humiliation she had been forced to undergo. In the end, the pain was relieved, albeit too late to save her life. For Kakima herself, although this was a crushing disappointment, deep down she was not surprised. For Sebati and Askhar it was the unkindest cut of all.

Askhar had already cared for his mother for many years. When the diagnosis of inoperable cancer was made, his devotion to her intensified. While she was in hospital, he visited daily from early morning until late at night. Sometimes, when she was especially distressed, he would sleep on a mattress on the floor. The brother and sister took turns feeding her, washing her, combing her thinning hair. They adorned the walls of her room with photos and memorabilia. There was a picture of Sebati as a 17-year-old girl when she won a beauty contest, with luscious, long, golden hair and a look of radiant happiness and confidence in the future. There was a photo of the children and their mother at the seaside during some holiday in the past. There were also religious objects, including a sign saying, perhaps a little provocatively, 'Trust Allah, Not Your Doctor'.

Sebati and Askhar saw themselves as their mother's carers and protectors. They prayed together with her in her room. They were her voice to the doctors and nurses. They scrutinised every aspect of her medical treatment and her nursing care, always insisting that the highest standards were maintained. On occasions, they felt compelled to point out deficiencies in the hospital procedures. Sometimes, this required a few sharp words, but these moments always passed quickly.

******

For an individual, the experience of suffering, grief or pain wells up as a particular form of engagement with the world. It induces a kind of disorientation, a loss of coordinates. The world that was previously concrete and fixed starts to appear contingent, uncertain, precipitous.

As a perturbation of the spatial and experiential boundaries of embodied experience, suffering opens up new insights. It blurs the boundaries of what seemed distinct and clear. It challenges the inner, physical economy of the senses and also the outer, social ones. Even if from the point of view of the individual undergoing it, suffering does not in itself have meaning, this relation to sense itself allows it to vary bodily and social experience and therefore to act as an organon of meaning.[5]

The person suffering can be strong or weak, brave or cowering, and those around her can also suffer. This is the case with Kakima and her family. They contemplate the anonymous and impersonal power that has taken over their lives. They are taken to the edge of meaning. Instead of a sense of benign plenitude, of satisfied completion, they find themselves facing an empty void, an indescribable horror of meaninglessness.

The reality of death is often encountered in this way, as an experience of a weakness in the face of an overpowering world. It is an experience of the horror of the absence of the world, of an absence of meaning in which all my abilities become unreal, until I myself disappear in its sombre passivity. The infinite passivity of dying is also the gradual closing of a future of unknown but open accomplishments. It is a suffering that does not pass away, can never become closed in either time or space. The passivity of death is therefore not just a condition that arises at the conclusion of life: it is always there at its boundaries. It is not just a distant, miraged end point: it permeates life from the beginning.

It is important not to conclude from this that the experiences of Kakima, Sebati and Askhar are merely echoes of those recorded over the ages. On the contrary, their suffering is novel, unique and singular. Kakima's experience of her illness and imminent death is hers alone. That which makes a person singular, what makes her *this* singular person, is not sayable. Sebati and Askhar decorate Kakima's hospital room in their own fashion, out of their own personal histories. The candles, the aromas, the music, the artefacts, the photos, the signs on the walls, the food: all of these evoke rich memories and experiences unique to the lifeworlds from which they have come.

Suffering breaches my individuality, as the passivity that gives rise to the presence of the other. It thereby also gives rise to the community of human beings dispersed into singular beings still dependent on each other. In this sense it is never entirely or exclusively my own. The true experience of suffering entails that it is not a solitary event. I am always concerned with the suffering of the other.[6]

Kakima's suffering is therefore both hers and at the same time it is not hers alone. Her pain opens up a cascade of reflections in all whom she touches: in Sebati, Askhar, and me. Instead of finding the ground of our own individuality, that which is properly ours and in regard to which we cannot be replaced, her travail exposes us to the dissipation of ourselves, to the experience of an insufferable anonymity. It opens us as individuals up to the suffering of other individuals. It makes possible our responses or understanding, of responsibility, or magnanimity.[7]

When Kakima, Sebati and Askhar look to me it is not for help but for understanding, and I know what they are asking. Kakima's sigh of resignation at the end of a long life of tempest and bitter struggle is perspicuous to me. The pathos of Sebati's and Askhar's devotion, the soft vulnerability beneath the harsh exterior, touches me deeply. I sense their fear, the desolation they are facing, the loss of the obdurate rock to which they have been secured.

******

No-one ever suffers alone. The other, suffering, turns to me. The surfaces of the other, surfaces of suffering, that face me appeal to me and make demands on me.[8] The other faces me, exposing to me the nakedness of his or her eyes, unshielded and unclothed. The other faces me with his or her words, which dissipate without leaving a trace and whose force I can resist by doing nothing.[9]

The cry of the one suffering always evokes a response of some kind, even if it is merely the response of pure recognition. However, recognition alone does not necessarily ease the pain. In Euripides' play *The Women of Troy*, quoted at the beginning of this chapter, Priam's wife Hecabe is a captive of the Greeks after the fall of Troy and the slaughter of the men. She is waiting with the other women to hear what will happen to them. To Hecabe's lament, the Chorus responds:

> Your cry of agony came to us, and we all
> Shuddered with nameless fears.

Hecabe can only reply with quietistic resignation:

> Let me lie. There's no comfort in your comforting,
> Here in the dust pain such as mine belongs—today's,
> Yesterday's, and tomorrow's pain ...[10]

What is it that locates for me 'the alien imperative on the surface of the other' that I see 'in the midst of the order of nature, of the practical field, and of society'?[11] It is the sense of this surface as a surface of suffering. In the face of the harsh contingency of the natural world, I encounter an imperative other than the laws of science, an imperative for an order beyond the finalities of the layout of things.

Suffering is one of the principal sources of ethics. It does not in itself have meaning but can generate meaning, shared meanings; that is, it is not a property of the individual sufferer. It is shared between us, immediately, primordially, as a condition of our mutual existence.[12] But it is more than this. Suffering as a shared experience is not just a common property of a multiplicity of consciousnesses. It does not reflect an 'altruistic' or 'caring' state of mind. The sharing itself is an expression of a foundational non-indifference, a responsibility, of one to another. It arises prior to any contract that would specify precisely the moment of reciprocity. In Levinas' words, 'The interhuman is also in the recourse that people have to one another for help, before the astonishing alterity of the other has been banalised or dimmed down to a simple exchange of courtesies'.[13]

******

But that is not quite how it happened in this case. Here, there was no magnanimity, on either side. At first, the hospital staff were touched by the family's devotion. Gradually, however, misgivings developed. They began to regard the children's refusal to accept their mother's inevitable death as importunate, even cruel. They attempted to move from active, life-sustaining therapy to symptom relief and palliation. Sebati and Askhar not only directly countermanded such a change but angrily accused the doctors of neglect and even negligence.

Sebati and Askhar spent even more time at the bedside, to offer their mother support and protection. A few weeks passed. By this time there was open hostility between Kakima's children on the one hand and the doctors and nurses on the other. The authorities decided to step in. There needed to be limits, they explained firmly. Visiting hours would be restricted. The orders of the doctors and the nurses had to be obeyed. The signs around the bed—'Trust Allah, Not Your Doctor'—had to be removed.

Sebati tried to ignore the new regulations but the hospital was intractable and advised that they were not negotiable. Sebati continued to ignore them. Staff removed the signs in the middle of the night. Sebati put them up again in the morning. The doctors and nurses became increasingly unsettled. They could see only the excess of the children's grief and grew alarmed when they realised that it could not be brought under control. The unfathomable emotion seemed irrational, the single-minded intensity increasingly terrifying and foreign.

There seemed to be no alternative. The authorities sought a court order to appoint an official guardian to make decisions regarding all aspects of Mrs Oqil's affairs. Sebati and Askhar were neither consulted nor represented. Expert witnesses were called. The family was criticised for acting against their mother's interests by rejecting medical advice. As expected, the court found in favour of the hospital and a guardian was appointed to take decision-making power away from Kakima and her children.

The guardian wasted no time. Within hours he had issued a range of injunctions. Kakima would be shifted to a nursing home. Sebati and Askhar were to be allowed to visit for only a few hours a day. They were not to feed their mother or to contribute to her care in other ways. They were not to take her on walks in a wheelchair. They were not to administer her herbal medicines. They were not to bring electronic devices or cameras into the hospital and they could be searched to ensure that they did not attempt to do so. There was to be no wailing and there could be no pictures on the walls or references to Allah. Praying would not be permitted.

Sebati and Askhar were incredulous, devastated. They felt betrayed and wronged. Sebati described the moment when she received the letter from the guardian, when she 'felt a sense of deep coldness piercing her heart'. She and Askhar were, after all, only doing their duty. Their cries, their mother's cries, it seemed, were being answered not with compassion but with poisonous hostility and vengeful bitterness.

Those who stood up for the patient—who included myself, her general practitioner and a few members of the staff—became the targets of the same hostility. On one occasion when I visited Mrs Oqil, I was advised that my role was regarded as that not of a doctor but of merely a friend, and the police were called to remove me from the hospital premises.

And what of Kakima? An old woman in a dry month waiting for rain. She was not consulted. The guardian did not visit her. No interpreters were called to help the staff or security guards seek her opinion. Her calls for her daughter and son to be beside her in her dying days went unheeded.

******

Not all cries for help are answered. Indeed, this is the age of cries for help denied. Every day, we turn away refugees. In Australia, people are allowed to drown as ships that could save them stand by, as happened on 19 October 2001 when the Australian Navy watched as 353 refugees died in the Timor Sea when a decrepit boat, code-named the SIEV X, capsized and sank. We invade and bomb other countries, directly or indirectly causing the death and injury of hundreds of thousands of civilians. We count our own dead but not those we kill. We ignore the needs of indigenous peoples, whose cultures are uprooted and dislocated by economic change, or of indigent people within our own borders suffering because of lack of adequate nutrition, shelter, education or health care.

It is hard to say if in the post-September 11 world, the post-Srebrenica, post-Iraq, post-Rwanda, post-Abu Ghraib, post-Guantanamo Bay world, there will be more denied, unacknowledged, unanswered cries from the suffering. It is hard to say if in the age of the War on Terror we have become crueller and less tolerant, whether imprisonment without trial, guilt by association or fear of other cultures is worse than it has been in earlier times.

Sebati and Askhar have obviously hit a raw nerve. Despite official commitment to cultural diversity and tolerance, the sheer intensity of their devotion to their mother and their grief at her illness throw out a deep challenge to the established system of care. Their raw emotion, their unfamiliar expressions of pain, disrupt the calm inevitability of institutional life. Their wild, uncontainable passion is experienced as darkly threatening, like the uproar in the jungle of Conrad's *Heart of Darkness*, where the black shapes crouch, lie, sit 'between the trees leaning against the trunks, clinging to the earth, half coming out, half effaced ... in all the attitudes of pain, abandonment, and despair'.[14]

******

But I, at least, am there to hear the cry. I am there to bear witness to Sebati's and Askhar's testimony, as I and others do to those of Anka, Pimbao and many others. I too discern the miscarriage of justice, the systematic cruelty of the system that punishes and criminalises those who cannot fathom their own suffering. I am dismayed by the irrationality and injustice of the system that claims to act in the name of reason and justice. But this is not so much a case of two truths coming into conflict with each other: rather, it is two untruths, two forms of unreason. This is not a clash of civilisations: it is a clash of abysses, of one species of unreason or incomprehension in intolerant opposition to another, equally implacable, equally uncompromising.

It is true that there is a radical difference between the suffering of the other—the testimony that he or she bears to the pain and the terror that shakes his or her body—and the reply to the call for help that arises in me as an external observer. I am the witness who can testify from afar, not with a detached, objective account, but as the one who affirms the experience of the patient and supplies it with meaning. The suffering in the other is unforgivable in me, solicits me and calls me, and suffers in me.

Why am I fascinated by suffering, I wonder to myself? Why do I travel across the world seeking it out? Why do I actively encourage sufferers to entrust me with their testimony? Is it out of a sense of personal guilt, that it is they who suffer and not I? I am troubled by the seductive attraction of the suffering of another, of the deep emotional power it exerts over me, and I am uncomfortable with the vicarious hallowedness acquired by contact with those who have personally suffered.

Am I drawn into the Oqils' predicament because of events in my own life, because my own parents are faltering too, because my own mother sadly, poignantly, also faces physical and mental decline, entering a new, touching innocence?[15] Is it because their story dramatises so poignantly my own imminent one, in which I too will be cut adrift from that which once sustained me? Am I witnessing my own mother's death, my own death? Why am I compelled to bear witness: to listen to the stories and record them? I am like the mother, Sebati's mother, my mother: I am the archive, the record of their personal histories, their hopes and their pain. I am compelled to listen, just as they are compelled to tell.

As Agamben has pointed out, the need to relate their stories was the force that kept many people alive during the Holocaust.[16] For some, like Primo Levi, once the story was told, the compulsion to continue living disappeared. But what does it do to you to witness suffering? What is the permanent mark, the stigma, that exposure to the pain of another leaves engraved on one's own life? Can any of us escape the private, enduring horror of Dr Managayam, the Sri Lankan doctor who heroically tended the wounded and the dying after the tsunami, who never left his post, for whom now, every time he closes his eyes, the terrible images of the victims well up viciously and accusingly before him?

******

Dr Managayam is compelled to relate his story again and again, in an attempt to depict experiences close to, or beyond, the edge of meaning. Philosophers, too, have attempted to provide meaning for such experiences. However, suffering is not a philosophical state and cannot be characterised according to a set of generic, universal principals. Its singularity is unique and irreducible. Even to attempt to describe it in language is to attenuate its meaning.

Attempts to describe suffering are thereby beset with a paradox. On the one hand, the need to give a voice to it is a condition of all truth, for suffering is an objective fact that weighs upon the subject. Its most subjective experience, its expression, is objectively conveyed.[17] On the other hand, rational cognition is unable to cope with suffering. It can never express it in the medium of experience, for to do so would be irrational by reason's own standards. There, even when it is understood, suffering remains mute and inconsequential.[18] That which this singular person experiences, that which makes me singular, is not sayable.

******

The conflict between Sebati and the authorities intensified and became even more acrimonious. The latter were evidently taken by surprise by the family's staying power and their dogged determination to fight back. In fact, from the family's point of view, they had no choice: they had to regain their mother's body, just like in many of the battles on the plains of Troy. They became increasingly frantic. Court battles were initiated, resulting in a long and bitter fight, much anxiety and many tears. Here, I was able to provide assistance, testifying to the commitment of Sebati and Askhar and to Mrs Oqil's own wishes.

In this fight, at least, we eventually achieved success. The guardianship order was lifted, a rare moment of triumph, and sombre celebration. The family felt vindicated. However, the triumph was short-lived. The conflicts with the professional health care system and the institutions, as it happened, were far from over.

Her authority renewed, Sebati proceeded to move her mother from one institution to another. Kakima's condition continued to deteriorate until she was barely conscious. Nonetheless, Sabati's demands for active investigation and treatment only became more insistent. Every day she demanded blood tests, new medical assessments, additional treatments. She and her brother remained at their mother's side, now between them maintaining an unrelenting 24-hour vigil. The care received at the hospital was never enough; the standards of nursing were always inadequate. Every time their mother's condition deteriorated, they demanded new treatments, fresh specialist assessments, additional blood tests, or maybe even a new hospital would be sought.

I talk with Mrs Oqil. It is the last conversation I will have with her. She makes clear that she trusts Sebati to make whatever decisions are necessary and states clearly that she herself has no particular requests. Nonetheless, even in her diminished state she continues ruthlessly to dominate her children. She demands to be fed, to be changed. She expects them to be there at all times, or, at least, this is their understanding of her expectations. Her expressions, her occasional words, are invariably interpreted as gestures or signs of disapproval. With time, however, she becomes weaker, loses the ability to speak at all, and lapses into silence.

I talk also with Sebati. I encourage her to acknowledge that her mother is dying. She has an incurable illness, I say. She herself is reconciled to her fate. You and Askhar have done your job admirably, but you have to accept that the process is inexorable, the end inevitable. Sebati becomes angry and forbids me ever again to talk in this way. Her mother will recover and will go home with her, she says. They will travel together. They will do things like in the old days, or rather things they had always said they would do. Did I not recognise that she was better today? She has surely turned the corner. Sebati has given up her business, her livelihood, to care for her mother. She would give her own heart if that would save her. Her mother lies silent and motionless. Sebati weeps convulsively.

Sebati and Askhar take their mother from one hospital to another—at last count, it has been eight in all. At each one the same pattern is repeated: the staff are at first touched by the devotion of the children and acquiesce to their demands, then they become diffident about the appropriateness of continued, burdensome treatment, then differences begin to surface with Sebati and Askhar, eventually degenerating into open hostility and an attempt to regulate their conduct with the help of security staff. Sebati and Askhar themselves follow their own fixed trajectory, resulting in each case in deepening anger and bitter recriminations.

******

Five months have passed since Kakima was admitted to hospital for what was thought to be the last stages of terminal care. Now in her eighth hospital, she is at best barely conscious. Sebati and Askhar are sitting by her bed, sponging her brow, adjusting her oxygen mask. The medical and nursing staff move in and out, perplexed, frustrated, seething. Sebati's anger is unabated.

The less Kakima is able to speak, the more vocal Sebati becomes. She writes me emails and sends text messages, sometimes many pages long. They often arrive in the middle of the night. The language is often opaque and obscure. She expresses her outrage at what she believes to be the inadequate care her mother has received. She blames everyone, accepts and forgives no-one. After such knowledge, she asks, what forgiveness is possible? She spends hours typing into the computer, in desperation, almost frenzy. The pain is palpable. Sometimes, there are just chains of single words or phrases: Outrage. Justice. Horror. Devastation. Obscure pain. Saturating darkness.

Her cry is shrill but poignant as it pierces the silence. Still her mother does not die.

The blank vastness of her sadness saps her strength, she writes. A horror, an amorphous, nameless horror, has engulfed their lives. When she heard that the doctors would no longer continue treatment, it was as if an explosion had gone off next to her and she was pierced by many shards of glass. She is angry at the doctors for abandoning her mother and at the nurses for their pretence at solicitude. The world seems to be floating, incoherent. No-one can understand—how could they, with the solid ground still under their feet?

Wild sorrow, dumb pain. Today, her mother is white as a ghost. Askhar is crying. There is a burst of yells, a whirl of limbs. Everything is blurred. She prays for those who have so much love to share. But it has been worth the pain. She just wants to live out her dreams and take her mama wherever she is led by Allah so she is able to heal her body and walk again. She is on the edge of the void, pierced to the heart.

She is an unpitied exile, old, her grey hair ravaged with the knife of mourning. The shadows are lengthening and soon the dark night will engulf all. There is pain in her marrow and bones. Woe rends her bosom apart. She moans, moans, moans and weeps to break her heart.

******

In her emails and text messages, Sebati strives to represent the unrepresentable, the timeless time and the spaceless space: the death of the mother who in reality had never been there for her. Her suffering is without present, just as it is without beginning or end. Time has radically changed its meaning and its flow; she is without past or future.

Despite all the words she pours out, despite all her cries, in reply Sebati can only hear silence. Silence is a word, a paradoxical word, that is linked to the cry, the voiceless cry, which breaks with all utterances, which is addressed to no-one and which no-one receives, the cry that lapses and decries. The cry does not simply come to a halt, reduced to nonsense. Yet it does remain outside of sense. It is a meaning infinitely suspended, decried, decipherable, indecipherable.

******

The stories of Kakima, Sebati and Askhar, and of Anka, Pimbao and Dr Managayam, are stories of deep pain, of bravery and heroism, of loss, of loyalty and commitment, of sacrifice, of the imperative to respond to the cries of others, of the impossibility of representing death, of the passivity, the contingency, the uncertainty and the irreducible singularity of suffering, of the black hole from which no meaning can escape but whose structures nevertheless found ethics. They are also stories of the power of testimony, of the 'equivocal, puzzling relation between words and voice', of the rhythm, melody, images, writing and silence that speak to us 'beyond ... words, beyond ... melody, like the unique performance of a singing'.[19]

When we tell stories of suffering in medical settings, we usually concentrate on intractable pain and loss. However, there are many features of suffering that are left out of this kind of account. Suffering is the direct experience of the world as contingent, fluid, uncertain. To suffer the world is to be both active and passive: the two must come together because openness to the world is not merely passive. Suffering does not have inherent meaning but through opening up new modalities at the edge of experience, it may become a route to knowledge. It is the boundary surface of the human world and that beyond.[20]

The pain continues and is inextinguishable. Suffering has no beginning and no end. At the end of her story, Hecabe cries softly:

> Who would not weep? City lost, children lost,
> All lost! Was there ever heard such chorus of pain?
> When were such tears shed for a murdered house?
> The chorus responds, on behalf of all of us:
> In times of sorrow it is a comfort to lament,
> To shed tears, and find music that will voice our grief.
> To this, the sombre reply follows, with resignation:
> The dead feel nothing; evil that can cause no pain.

> But one who falls from happiness to unhappiness
> Wanders bewildered in a strange and hostile world.[21]

******

After seven months of suffering, Mrs Oqil finally died, with Sebati and Askhar at her side. When the end came, she had been unconscious for two weeks. Sebati was as devastated as if the death had occurred suddenly, without warning. She lamented her guilt at having slept that night, complaining that she had been robbed of precious hours with her mother. She blamed herself for her mother's death, saying that if she had only given her more or better food, or other medicines, or had been more insistent with the doctors, things might have been different.

Askhar was numbed but reflected quietly. Now the turmoil was over, he was concerned that some might accuse him and his sister of prolonging their mother's suffering. That was not it at all, he says. He was just doing his duty, even if that duty seems a little less clear from the present vantage point. He had remained at his post to the end. He spoke softly about the impending change in his life, which might even include marriage.

The day of the funeral is stiflingly hot. Sebati and Askhar are transfixed and motionless as the body is lowered into the deep grave and the men set to work with their shovels, turning up clouds of choking dust. When they have finished, Sebati, barely audible, describes the first night without her mother. It has been the darkest, cruellest night of her life. A blackness has come over her world, submerging her, saturating her, covering everything, including all she had known and cared for. Her mother had been a rich jewel in a cruel, barren, harsh world. The grave has been filled but the eternal hole will always gape. A dead tree gives no shelter and the dry stone no sound of water.

She finishes by expressing her gratitude to me for the support I have given and asks me to say some words. I thank her, saying how privileged I have been to be able to witness the family's loyalty and courage and the intensity of their love. When I have finished, I go back to my car, alone, for the drive home, and I weep.

Notes

1. Euripides, *The Women of Troy*, tr. P Vellacott (London, Penguin, 1973), p. 93.
2. D Leder, *The Absent Body* (Chicago, University of Chicago Press, 1990), p. 73.
3. J-P Sartre, *Being and Nothingness*, tr. H Barnes (New York, Washington Square Press, 1971), p. 438.
4. E Levinas, 'Useless Suffering', in *Entre Nous*, trs M Smith and B Harshaw (New York, Columbia University Press, 1988), p. 93.
5. There is nothing remarkable about this. The same can be said about many other modalities of bodily experience, including illness in general.
6. M Blanchot, *The Unavowable Community*, tr. P Joris (New York, Station Hill Press, 1988), p. 21.
7. L Irigaray, *An Ethics of Sexual Difference*, trs C Burke and GC Gill (New York, Cornell University Press, 1993), p. 151: 'We need to return to the moment of prediscursive experience, recommence everything, all the categories by which we understand things, the world, subject–object divisions, recommence everything and pause at the mystery as familiar as it is unexplained, of a light which, illuminating the rest, remains at its source in obscurity'.
8. A Lingis, *The Community of Those Who have Nothing in Common* (Bloomington, Indiana University Press, 1994), p. 32.
9. ibid.
10. Euripides, *The Women of Troy*, p. 106.
11. A Lingis, *The Community of Those Who Have Nothing in Common*, p. 29.
12. E Levinas, 'Useless Suffering', p. 94.
13. ibid., p. 101.
14. J Conrad, *Heart of Darkness* (New York, Bantam Books, 1960), p. 24.
15. J Derrida, *Demeure: Fiction and Testimony*, tr. E Rottenberg (Stanford, Stanford University Press, 2000), p. 43: 'In essence a testimony is always autobiographical: it tells, in the first person, the sharable and unsharable secret of what happened to me, to me to me alone, the absolute secret of what I was in a position to live, see, hear, touch, sense, and feel'.
16. G Agamben, *Remnants of Auschwitz* (New York, Zone Books, 1999), p. 15.
17. T Adorno, *Negative Dialectics*, tr. EB Ashton (London, Routledge and Kegan Paul, 1973), p. 17.
18. T Adorno, *Aesthetic Theory*, tr. C Lenhardt (London, Routledge and Kegan Paul, 1984), p. 27.
19. S Felman and D Laub, *Crises of Witnessing in Literature, Psychoanalysis and History* (New York, Routledge, 1992), pp. 277–8.
20. J Derrida, *Demeure: Fiction and Testimony*, pp. 25ff.
21. Euripides, *The Women of Troy*, pp. 110–11.

CHAPTER 11

How to End a Life

I am going to tell the story of the death of a man I never knew. Mr Bravic died six weeks after I met him—or rather, saw him, since we were never able to exchange words.

In clinical practice, there is a logic—the logic of biology and disease—and this is what doctors utilise. However, individual lives, the experience of illness, the course of disease, cannot be contained within this logic. The illness typically precipitates a process that far exceeds the cause, that resonates throughout the lifeworld not only of the individual concerned but also much more widely, to include the whole social and cultural setting in which she conducts her life.

As Deleuze has shown, an individual is a multiplicity, the actualisation of a set of virtual singularities that function together, that enter into symbiosis, that attain a certain consistency. It—the individual—is in a state of becoming, not just in the sense that it does not have a static being and is in constant flux, but also because there is an objective zone of indistinction or indiscernibility between any two multiplicities, a zone that immediately precedes their respective natural differentiation. In a multicentred world, a multiplicity is defined not by its centre but by the limits and borders where it enters into relation with other multiplicities, changes its nature and transforms itself.

In opposition to the common assumptions of doctors and bioethicists, the processes of clinical causality are complex.[1] Events cannot be reduced to their biological, psychological, or social conditions. Corporeal causality in particular is not complete.[2] Something always occurs that cannot be properly described at the level of corporeal causes and effects. To use Deleuzian language again: Becoming cannot be reduced to Being; we need always to consider together the molar and the molecular, the Nomadic and the State.

The job of the clinician is to work within the dynamics of the multiplicity, to follow its lines of force, to seek to construct sense through language, often in the midst of chaos and dissolution of meaning.[3]

******

One Sunday evening—it was a hot day in January—I was called by the Intensive Care Unit (ICU) consultant on duty to provide assistance with a difficult problem that had developed in the unit. He described the clinical background in a few brief words. The problem was simple: the patient, Frank Bravic, was unconscious and had no hope of surviving, but his wife, Rosa, would not allow the machines keeping him alive to be turned off.

I came to ICU and reviewed the history with the doctors and nurses. The patient, in his early fifties, was awaiting a heart transplant. He had been sick for years. Many people die on the waiting list because there are too few organs. His condition deteriorated and he was about to die. They inserted a mechanical left ventricular assist device—an 'LVAD'.

The LVAD is a device as big as a washing machine that has tubes and cords running in and out of it. It is attached to the heart and so-called great vessels. It pumps the blood, keeps it flowing. It is not a cure, only a temporary measure to keep the heart going until someone dies and his or her heart becomes available for transplantation.

Mr Bravic had his LVAD installed and he felt immediately better. He was from all accounts very optimistic. When later, hours before his death, Rosa recounted the course of events to me, she recalled that everything had gone well for a few days. Everyone laughed and joked about it. His family called him 'machine man'. He was even planning to go home. There was a sense of euphoria, of unreality. The sense of unreality, as it turned out, was well justified.

One of the requirements of an artificial device such as this is that the propensity of the blood to clot be prevented. Accordingly, an anticoagulant is administered to stop the blood clotting in the artificial environment. With this treatment there is a risk of haemorrhage—that is, excessive bleeding—which can sometimes be disastrous.

That's exactly what happened in Mr Bravic's case. On the seventh day after installation of the LVAD, disaster struck. He suffered a large bleed into his brain. He never regained consciousness in the two months he lived after that.

It was a devastating shock to everyone. The doctors were disappointed. It had seemed such a good result, but now the outlook seemed very bleak. If recovery were to occur at all, the damage would be very extensive. Certainly, a heart transplant was now permanently off the agenda.

The ICU doctors took Rosa aside and broke the bad news to her. There was no hope. It was very sad. The machine was intended only as a temporary measure pending transplantation. Because this was no longer possible, it would be necessary to withdraw treatment. She was incredulous. It was not possible, not comprehensible. She refused to give permission for the machines to be turned off. The carers understood. They had been there before, many times. They knew how difficult it was. She would be given a couple of days and the subject would be broached again.

******

In medicine, as in capitalism, individuals are understood as freely exchangeable units. These units are seen as essentially the same or at least reducible to the same. In such a world, the relations between people are thought of only as those between similar units: all are the same and can be exchanged for one another. That is why today we no longer speak of an ethical community, but merely about morally controlled marketplaces of human objectification.[4]

******

The days went by and Rosa did not change her stance. She could not give permission for treatment to be discontinued.

******

I met Rosa for the first time that Sunday night in the relatives' room outside the ICU itself. This room is claustrophobic and a bit stifling. It has two doors: one passes out to the waiting room, which is usually full of tearful or solemn relatives sitting with vacant expressions, waiting for the hours to pass; the other, protected by a security key pad, leads to the ICU. There are no windows. The chairs are vinyl and steel, a few too many for the space. The smell is of disinfectants and those indefinable sweet chemical odours that we associate with hospitals.

I introduced myself and explained my role. I emphasised that I was not there to represent the hospital and had no view about what course of action should be taken.

It's true: I have no bias; I am not representing anyone. I am there to talk and to help negotiate. I am, in this role, no-one's advocate, and nor am I a physician. My job is to help the parties sort out the meanings inherent in their predicament. But what if there are none? What if we have passed the limits of sense? After all, I already know that there is no hope, that Mr Bravic will die despite anything that may be said or done.

I am familiar with the incredulity and dissolution of sense that often accompanies the illness or death of a loved one: the sense of inexorability and of chaos. Once, in dire circumstances, a patient's husband absently quoted to me Macbeth's words, as if he were inventing them himself. 'Life's but a walking shadow', he said, 'a poor player'

> That struts and frets his hour upon the stage
> And then is heard no more: it is a tale
> Told by an idiot, full of sound and fury,
> Signifying nothing.[5]

******

Rosa is suspicious and hostile. They are trying to kill her husband. It is a conspiracy. She cannot leave him alone for a moment. She must scrutinise their every move, read the labels on the vials of medication they inject into him, check that the machines continue to operate, remind them to turn him, change his dressings.

The hospital is supposed to be a secure environment, a place where you can trust that you will be cared for, a place of hope. Instead, for her, it is a hell, a place of uncertainty and threat.

I buy time. I talk with her and ask if I can see her again. She is unwilling to talk much, and her sentences are terse and sometimes brutal. I assure her, without qualification, that she can trust me. I will not let her down. I give her my word. We keep meeting. I sit with her for long periods, often with few words passing between us. Gradually, she accepts my role and, however tentatively, begins to talk. I give her my mobile number and tell her she can call me any time. When from time to time she does so, I am pleased. She calls with concerns that have come up in the ward. I make a point of coming in unfailingly to the hospital to sort them out.

She tells me about their life together—not so much about herself, really, but mainly about Frank. He had his faults, but she stood by him. There were hard times. Nothing dramatic. There was no great passion, no exciting adventures, just a mundane shared life.

******

Frank had come from Hungary thirty-three years before. He was nineteen. It was just after the liberalisation started in the 1960s and he took the first chance to leave. He got off the plane penniless, with little education and no skills. A few months later, Rosa arrived. I never found out how it was that she travelled across the world, alone, at the age of sixteen.

In one of the few times I saw her smile, Rosa described their first meeting. She was shy and embarrassed. He was callow, but handsome and imposing. They fell in love at once and were married within a couple of months. It was a struggle after that. She worked in factories and in a shop. He worked as a storeman, a builder, a factory hand. They saved a bit of money, but didn't make it big. There were hard times, but they stuck by one another.

She matured within their love. They had two children. Their relationship was not without problems, but there was undoubted deep loyalty and unquestioning commitment. Indeed, as I reflected to myself while listening to her, not many people have the privilege of loving, or being loved, like that.

******

Rosa continued her story in a somewhat disjointed but nonetheless compelling way. When Frank became sick, he did not give any thought to dying. He never mentioned it. The family never discussed it. Rosa was always there when he saw the doctors. She was no fool. On the contrary, she was articulate and strong. She had come to speak English better than her native tongue.

When Frank's illness was discussed, she was always at his side. She listened and took part. She could not remember any discussions about the possibility of a bad outcome, either in the medical consultations or within the family. She could not recall a single mention of death.

******

For an individual, death is the horror of the absence of the world, of an absence of meaning in which all my abilities become unreal, until 'I' myself disappear in the passivity in dying. In the process of dying, one is exposed to the possibility of an existence deprived of the world of action. In such existence, the idea of authentic death, as the origin of my knowledge, is transformed into the infinite passivity of dying, where the one who dies encounters the impossibility of dying; that is to say, the impossibility of turning the world into something meaningful.

Although it is always a solitary experience, death is never my own, and it never belongs just to someone else. I am always implicated in the death of the other.[6] Death as breaching my individuality, death as the passivity that gives rise to the presence of the other, also gives rise to the community of human beings dispersed into singular beings still dependent on each other.

The knowledge of death is the specifically human tragedy. Except for human beings, all animals live in immortality, for they are ignorant of death. What is 'divine, terrible, incomprehensible, is to know that one is immortal'. As Jorge Luis Borges has expressed it,

> Death (or its allusion) makes men precious and pathetic. They are moving because of their phantom condition; every act they execute may be their last; there is not a face that is not on the verge of dissolving like a face in a dream. Everything among ... mortals has the value of the irretrievable and the perilous.[7]

Humans have to earn, gain, construct their immortality. Or at least they used to. With the advent of a range of new technologies—computers, video cameras, CD writers and the rest—immortality, at least in a weakened, attenuated sense, has become a readily available commodity. In hospitals, too, people can be conjoined with machines that keep their hearts beating, that keep their lungs moving, long after they would have succumbed to the disease process that precipitated initiation of treatment.[8]

Some say that death itself has been degraded too by the unrestrained proliferation of images about death, by the daily presentation of dying children or bleeding civilians in our living rooms. This banalisation of mass, anonymous death contrasts with the traditional annulment of individual death, which continues to be hidden in hospitals and banned from public discourse.

This process has, of course, been extensively discussed over the last half-century. Indeed, the deconstruction of death has been one of the main concerns of modernity. In our postmodern times, it is perhaps the turn of immortality to be deconstructed. Do the new technologies of health and information efface the opposition between death and immortality, between the transitory and the durable?[9] Do they transform modern citizens into strange postmodern simulacra, into mechanical and electronic equivalents of the picture of Dorian Gray?

******

The days went by. As foretold, there was no discernible improvement in Frank. For Rosa and her family, this was excruciating. The doctors daily sought to disconnect the machines, to let him die. But they needed her agreement. They tried different strategies: at one time, they were kind and cajoling; at another, they were firm and insistent. They reasoned with her. They pleaded with her. There were others, they said, with greater need for the bed. It was sad, they told her, but life must move on.

But she was obdurate. She would not give up. She remained at his bedside night and day. She held his hand and whispered to him. She sponged his face. She stroked him—as Marguerite Duras put it—'as if he ran the risk of happiness'.[10]

For her, there was nothing beyond her life with Frank. No future could be contemplated without him. She seemed to understand what was being said, but it was as if it was her own death they were discussing. At times, the discussions became acrimonious. In response to their veiled threats to act without her consent, she tersely advised them that if they disregarded her wishes she would take legal action. They wrote in the history that she exhibited paranoid behaviour. She experienced chest pains and paid a visit herself to the Emergency Department.

But her adamantine resolve did not alter. She wouldn't give permission. She could not allow her husband to die.

******

I talk with the doctors. We need to care for her. She will be the survivor. She suffers as much as he does. Rosa is our patient now.

More time goes past. Unexpectedly, Frank starts to improve. She notices it before anyone else. At first they say she is just imagining it, that it is a sign of her desperation. But it soon becomes apparent that she is right. He begins to wake up. He opens his eyes and recognises Rosa and the children. He smiles at them and plays with his daughter's hair the way he used to do.

The family is exultant. Rosa in particular is vindicated, triumphant. Her loyalty has borne fruit. Her prayers have been answered. They weep tears of joy. They notify all their friends. Many come to see him. They bring flowers and suddenly Frank's room, until now a site of lachrymose despair, is filled with music and colour. There are smiles of magnanimity and quiet satisfaction.

But the doctors, however disconcerted by the unexpected turn of events, make no concessions. After all, they have the weight of the laws of nature on their side. His underlying condition, they point out, remains perilous. The improvement, they warn darkly, can only be ephemeral.

At first, this seems ungracious and pusillanimous. But sadly, and too quickly, they are proved correct. The very next day Mr Bravic suffers a further stroke. He subsides into deep unconsciousness. This time, there will be no return.

Rosa is doubly devastated. She admits that he no longer responds. Now the bad news comes fast. He has infections. His lungs are deteriorating. His liver function is declining. His kidneys are starting to fail.

Her pain is deep, her despair unfathomable. The sight is dismal. Death feasts in its eternal cell.

******

Rosa and I become closer. The ideology of medical practice is that it favours reason and cognition over emotion and intuition. However, a therapeutic relationship—or any relationship for that matter—is unthinkable in the absence of an ethical dimension. This ethical relationship, furthermore, is not grafted on to an antecedent relationship of cognition. Rather, as Levinas points out, it is a foundation and not a superstructure.[11] This is especially true for a relationship of which the sole rationale is ethical discourse:

> Outside of the hunger one satisfies, the thirst one quenches, and the senses one allays, exists the other, absolutely other, desired beyond these satisfactions, when the body knows no gesture to slake the desire, where it is not possible to invent any new caress. The desire is unquenchable, not because it answers to an infinite hunger, but because it does not call for food.[12]

But let us not forget Frank. He himself has receded from view, become indistinct. From a medical point of view, there is (and despite the brief, bittersweet moment of resurrection, there has been) no hope. He has become merged with the machine that has taken over his vital functions. He is a machine attached to a machine. The relentless pounding of the mechanical pump is at once his own body and a foreign contrivance. It has long become unclear where his biological tissues end and the inorganic organs begin. The categories, which once seemed obvious, of the natural and factitious, of the human and the mechanical, have become blurred. Similarly, the tragic fragility of his body, with the precarious mortality that has been the focus of his medical treatment, has given way to the inexorable, indestructible logic of the machine that dwells inside him.

Of course, in a sense, we are all continuous with machines—we are all in some sense cyborgs. In this case, however, it is not just that Mr Bravic dwells within the technology. He *is* the machine. Thus, the grotesque logic of the technology generates a double irony. With it, his body, which has otherwise lost its ability to sustain itself, pounds on, indestructible. But technology or no technology, his alterity perdures. A gap opens up between the tremulous insubstantiality of his unaided physical body and the potent constancy of the social lifeworlds in which he is embedded.

A person's identity is tied to the system of signs constituted by the network of his social relations. Attaching him to a machine is an operation on the production of sense: it changes the understanding of, and the meanings attached to, his body and it instrumentalises both the physical body and its social relationships. As the biological control systems that define his material body continue to disintegrate, he is reduced to no more than a cipher, a trope in a disembodied universe of signs.

There is a logic to the circulation of signs in the contemporary world that is very familiar. Words and images proliferate within multiple semiotic systems, not arborially as in a centralised factory, but rhizomatically, at any decentred location. As Baudrillard said, 'The signs evolve, they concatenate and produce themselves, always one upon the other—so that there is no basic reference which can sustain them'.[13]

The superimposition of radical biotechnologies, however, adds yet another element. As Slavoj Zizek put it in explicitly Deleuzian language, the productive flux of pure becoming that defined the body without organs, the body not yet structured or determined as functional organs, gives way to the organs without a body; that is, to the virtuality of pure affect extracted from its embeddeness in the body. The virtual as the site of productive becoming is supplanted by the virtual as the site of the sterile sense event. What is left is no more than an uncanny trace of what was once palpable and pulsating, like the slowly fading smile of a Cheshire cat.[14] In the end, however, even the smile disappears.

If the logic of biotechnology is to generate a new species of immortality, what are the conditions for controlling mortality today? How is the gap between the tremulous, ephemeral, private body and the stridency of the semiotic systems to be closed?

******

The answer is, no doubt, the same as it has always been. Immortality exists ultimately only in the symbolic realm. Therefore, deletion of the corporeal schema cannot itself fill the gap. What is needed is a resymbolisation of the lifeworld. This is the task of the process of grieving, classically described by Freud:

> Reality testing has shown that the loved object no longer exists, and it proceeds to demand that all libido shall be withdrawn from its attachments to that object. This demand arouses understandable opposition—it is a matter of general observation that people never willingly abandon a libidinal position, not even, indeed, when a substitute is already becoming available to them. This opposition can be so intense that a turning away from reality takes place and a clinging to the object through the medium of a hallucinatory wishful psychosis ... [T]he existence of the lost object is psychically prolonged ... [W]hen the work of mourning is completed the ego becomes free and uninhibited again.[15]

Successful mourning, however, does not entail merely the loosening of the ties to the loved object and the possibility of replacing it by another. To be successful, there needs to be a process of self-transformation, an enigmatic process of loss accompanied by searching and rediscovery. This rediscovery, furthermore, always contains some recognition of our fundamental, ethical interdependence on others, of our crucial, but impossible, insertion in community. Grief is not, as is often assumed, a private, solitary experience that cuts us off from all other people. On the contrary, what grief displays is 'the thrall in which our relations with others hold us', in ways that we cannot always recount or explain, in ways that often interrupt the self-conscious accounts of ourselves we try to provide, that challenge the very notion of ourselves as autonomous and in control.[16]

The body implies mortality, vulnerability, agency: the skin and the flesh expose us to the gaze of others, but also to touch, and to violence, and bodies put us at risk of becoming the agency and instrument of these as well. Constituted as a social phenomenon in the public sphere, my body is and is not mine.[17] What calls me into question most radically is not the sheer ephemeralness of my physical existence but my presence for another who absents himself by dying.[18] Indeed, this is the only separation that can open me, in its very impossibility, to the openness of a community. To experience loss, to be with someone who is dying, perhaps more than anything else exposes the ethical foundations of all human relationships. This is the—paradoxical—'gift of death', about which George Bataille spoke with such poignancy:

> [B]y dying, you not only remove yourself, you are also present, for here you grant me that dying like a granting that surpasses all suffering, and here I tremble softly in my tears, losing speech even as you do, dying with you without you, letting myself die in your place, receiving the gift beyond you and me.[19]

In this sense, death is at the foundation of all community, of all ethical responsibility. Both death and ethics entail the presentation of our mortal truth, of our finitude and excess. Both present, simultaneously, the darkest threat and the most unfathomable promise.

******

The signs continued to proliferate. It had been a long two weeks. Mr Bravic had been kept alive at huge expense to provide an opportunity for Rosa to come to terms with what had been inevitable from the beginning. He had received extensive treatment and support with no limitation, even though his physical life had effectively ended weeks ago.

Rosa had no doubt worked hard. But so had the nurses who had laboured over the failing body with the treatments and the machines: feeding, cleaning, turning, monitoring, adjusting. They were very perplexed by their personal predicament. After all, whom were they treating? Was it Mr Bravic or his wife? For weeks they had laboured to keep alive a corpse, in the hope that his wife could survive. The actual body they were tending had ceased to be sustainable, but it is surely not the role of the ICU to sustain virtual bodies, however replete with meaning they may remain.

The ICU doctors too were anxious: was this not a profligate, irresponsible waste of the community's resources? After all, it was costing $10 000 a day to sustain him. The patient had been accorded his proper dignity. Were there not other, now more worthy, patients requiring our attention? Should we not now move on to the next interchangeable cipher to take Mr Bravic's place?

Both Frank and Rosa had been given their chance, but the die had rolled the wrong way. Now, something had to be done. Even if Mr Bravic was immortal at a symbolic level, his ravaged body ultimately was not. The relentless pulsing of the machine can go on forever. But it can also be switched off. That is what had to happen.

******

Rosa trusted me. She had said things to me she had never before said to anyone. Gradually, grudgingly, she came to concede that her husband could not survive.

Slowly, she became convinced that the ICU doctors were right: that the fact that his heart or lungs worked at all was merely an artefact of the mechanical device. Without it, he would die immediately. He could not, he would not, survive.

At last, she accepted the inevitable. In abject despair, she agreed that treatment should be discontinued. The heart-assist device would be turned off and her husband allowed to die. She thanked me wanly for the support I had given and praised my patience and kindness. We were all gratified in our own sadness, and proud of our achievement. It had, after all, been a difficult and challenging experience for us too. We congratulated the family on their courage and suggested that they say a last farewell. They did so, and with profound and silent sorrow they retired to the relatives' room while the machine was inactivated.

******

But endings are never happy. Switching off the machine turned out not to be easy, frustrated by multiple backup power sources and failsafe devices. In our desperation, we removed batteries and disconnected wires and cables. Eventually, the machine was disabled and grudgingly ground to a halt.

We watched and waited. To our surprise and horror, Mr Bravic did not die. His own lungs—so damaged—kept breathing. His own heart—so ravaged—kept beating. Ten minutes, twenty, thirty, forty minutes went by. The family had said their goodbyes and were waiting outside to receive final confirmation of his demise. We had to tell them that despite disconnection from the machine, he had not succumbed immediately as we had predicted.

Panic and shock, howls and hopeless despair. Shouts and tears, unspeakable, unfathomable pain. Everyone is reeling. Tongues and hearts cannot conceive or name the horror. Rosa staggers and falls. She is helped to her feet and supported by her son and daughter. More shrieks and piercing lamentations: a scene of woeful desolation. I go to comfort Rosa. She pushes me aside. She screams: 'Get away from me! I trusted you! You betrayed me!'

Mr Bravic died two hours later. Rosa did not speak to me again. The family left the hospital and returned home interstate that night. They did not thank the hospital before they left. We wrote a nice letter expressing our sympathy. We never received a reply.

Notes

1   See A Lingis, *Excesses: Eros and Culture* (Albany, State University of New York Press, 1983).
2   G Deleuze and F Guattari, *A Thousand Plateaus: Capitalism and Schizophrenia*, tr. Brian Massumi (Minneapolis, University of Minnesota Press, 1987), pp. 149–66; S Zizek, *Organs without Bodies: Deleuze and Consequences* (New York, Routledge, 2004), p. 27.
3   G Deleuze, 'What is Multiplicity?', in *The Deleuze Reader*, ed. CV Boundas (New York, Columbia University Press, 1993), chapters 4, 15.
4   M Blanchot, *The Unavowable Community*, tr. P Joris (New York, Station Hill Press, 1988) p. 102.
5   W Shakespeare, *Macbeth* (Cambridge, Cambridge University Press, 1947), Act V, Scene V.
6   M Blanchot, *The Unavowable Community*, p. 21.
7   JL Borges, *Labyrinths* (Middlesex, Penguin, 1964), pp. 144, 146.
8   Z Bauman, *Postmodernity and Its Discontents* (New York, New York University Press, 1997), p. 163.
9   ibid., p. 161.
10 M Duras, *The Malady of Death* (Canada, Grove Press, 1986).
11 E Levinas, *Collected Philosophical Papers*, tr. A Lingis (Dordrecht, The Netherlands, Nijhoff, 1987), p. 56.
12 ibid.
13 J Baudrillard, 'The Evil Demon of Images', in *Baudrillard Live: Selected Interviews*, ed. M Gane (London, Routledge, 1993), p. 141.
14 S Zizek, *Organs without Bodies*, p. 55.
15 S Freud, 'Mourning and Melancholia', in S Freud, *The Complete Psychological Works*, Volume XIV, tr. L Strachey (London, The Hogarth Press, 1974), p. 244.

16 J Butler, *Precarious Life* (London, Verso, 2004), p. 22.
17 ibid., p. 26.
18 M Blanchot, *The Unavowable Community*, p. 9.
19 ibid. The passage continues: 'To which there is this answer: "In the illusion that makes you live while I am dying." To which there is this answer: "In the illusion which makes you die while you die."'

Chapter 12

Fardels of the Heart
Obesity and the Unbearable Heaviness of Being

> And send us prying into the abyss,
> To gather what we shall be when the frame
> Shall be resolved to something less than this
> Its wretched essence;
> It is enough in sooth that once we bore
> These fardels of the heart—the heart whose sweat was
>   gore.[1]

Health problems related to excessive weight or obesity have acquired major importance in modern Western societies. In Australia, it is said that nearly two-thirds of people are overweight and about one-third are obese. A long list of health problems is attributed to or associated with excessive weight, and the economic cost is said also to be great.

Both the causes of the high prevalence of obesity and the most appropriate responses to it are the subject of intense debate. The causes appear to include increased availability and aggressive marketing of convenience foods, processed foods of high-energy density, increased use of motor cars, automation in the workplace and increased time spent in passive entertainment pursuits.

The responses to this modern plague include a search for new pharmaceutical treatments, and public health campaigns directed towards encouraging people to reduce their energy intakes and to exercise more. There has been a huge increase in commercial enterprises selling medical therapies and weight loss programs, even though the evidence shows that these are at best minimally effective. Additional measures under consideration include banning food advertising and marketing to children, imposing food and physical activity requirements on schools, and controlling the availability of convenience foods and drinks.

While obesity may well be associated with significant and increasing health problems, there are key assumptions that are often overlooked. One major gap is the absence of voices of the people living with obesity themselves. This chapter is a contribution to redressing this lacuna.

My understanding and insights are derived from my conversations with many of my patients, one in particular, whom I will call 'Jo'. Before I proceed further, therefore, I would like to introduce her to you.

******

Although Jo was only thirty-eight when I met her a couple of years ago, she had already had a long life. What struck me from the very first was her deep sense of sadness and tiredness. She had spent a lifetime battling weight issues, medical problems, family conflicts and financial worries. All she wanted, she said, was to be able to rest and be happy.

When she was growing up, Jo had thought of herself as an ordinary kid. The family lived in the western suburbs of their home city; they weren't well off but they weren't poor either. It was not a close family. Her parents' marriage was unhappy and sometimes marred by her father's violent behaviour. There was little sharing of emotion. In fact, Jo reflected that she never saw either of her parents cry, and she felt that neither of them was ever aware of the personal pain and suffering she endured.

It was not until puberty, when she started putting on weight, that she began to think of herself as different. Whether it was her weight that separated her from her classmates or her sense of being different that led to her weight gain, she could not decide. However, her memories of high school were dominated by a sense of alienation and exclusion, and sometimes frank humiliation. What she experienced then continued throughout her entire life.

When she was sixteen, her weight was already 80 kg and by the age of twenty it was 100 kg. it continued to increase inexorably, especially after her pregnancies. By the time she was thirty she weighed 160 kg, and on her thirty-ninth birthday she registered 203 kg. The extreme weight ravaged her body: she suffered from diabetes, heart disease, severe breathing problems and painful arthritis, and could walk only with great difficulty, with the help of two sticks.

******

Jo and I talked at length about her struggle, her hopes and deep fears, and her body. We talked about what it is like to live within an obese body. Of course, this is a bad way to put it. I experience my body not primarily as an object among others in the world, or as a thing that I occupy. Rather, I am embodied, in the sense that I live my body, not just that I have one.[2] My lived body is just not an objective, physiological body. It is rather the condition and context through which I am able to have relations with objects. My body is immanent and transcendent. I live it, as it is experienced by me. It provides the horizon that establishes my place in the world and makes possible my relations with other people and other things.

My body is my being in the world. It is the means by which I obtain knowledge and generate meaning. It constitutes the field within which I establish my cohesion and identity as a subject, the basic schema of orientation, the centre of my systems of coordinates.[3] My body, therefore, is not the means by which I experience the world; it is not a mere property of my personality or individuality; it is not a collection of organs and tissues subject to health and disease. At least, it is not just these things: it is also who I am and how I exist in the world. It defines and shapes my self-representations, my sources of sensuous pleasure and my relationships with others.

My body is private: indeed, it is the very meaning of private. It is also my link to other bodies. My flesh is not a pure object: it is a component of the medium within which I interact with others and set my personal course.[4] Different meanings are made possible through fluctuations or perturbations in the bodily schema. It is not just a matter of meaning either: the mutated manifold transforms the very conditions of knowledge and experience.

There has been extensive discussion about the lived experience of the sick body[5], the sexed body[6], and the disabled body.[7] To take the last example, Kay Toombs has written about the experiences of people with disabilities, drawing on her own experience of multiple sclerosis. She describes in detail the disruption of the lived body engendered by the loss of mobility. This includes a change in the character of surrounding space, an alteration in one's taken-for-granted awareness of (and interaction with) objects, the disruption of corporeal identity, a disturbance in one's relations with others, and a change in the character of temporal experience. The loss of upright posture is of particular significance since it not only concretely diminishes autonomy but affects the way in which one is treated by others.[8]

What about the lived experience of the obese body? I will let Jo speak in her own words:

> My body feels alien to me. It is as if it is not my own any more. When I was a girl I was nimble and lithe. I loved dancing and I was the fastest runner in the class. I was always running everywhere. They couldn't stop me. Now it is painful for me even to stand up from sitting. I have to use two sticks to walk. Even the simplest daily tasks require effort. Sometimes it is too much to be worth it. I can't sit in most chairs. I haven't gone to a movie in years.
>
> Everything I experience is through the lens of my fat. I once looked up 'heavy' in the dictionary and found that almost all the terms applied to me: my body is slow, obdurate, ponderous, cumbersome, lumpish, ungraceful, oppressive, stodgy, inert.
>
> When I go to Target to buy a T-shirt the shop girl looks me up and down with undisguised contempt. When I go to the doctor for a Pap smear I sense his revulsion as he approaches me, lying on the couch. I try to shrink away, to look small. I imagine my liquid fat dribbling down the legs of the couch, forming an embarrassing, filthy puddle on the floor of his spotless surgery.
>
> Sometimes I try to imagine my body to be a kind of thin body, bigger than most, but able to pass as thin. I try to block out my bulges, rolls and dimples, my fleshy spillages. I try not to look at myself in mirrors or shop windows.

I bind myself up in elastic underwear, wrap myself in dark colours, trying to hide my body from myself and from the gazes of others.[9]

In public, no matter what I wear, I feel naked. I can see what people are thinking. The first thought that passes through their heads when they look at me is 'fat'. Last week I was in the train and someone exclaimed loudly to his companion so that I could hear, 'The trouble with fat people is that they take up too much space!'

In the supermarket people standing next to me in the queue always scrutinise what I buy. I always buy good food now—much better than most. I only eat organic food and I am a vegetarian. I have watched every morsel, counted every calorie, that has gone into my mouth since I was 16. I don't eat MacDonald's or drink Coca Cola. But I can see what they are thinking: 'She is a glutton. She lacks control. I bet she'll eat all that tonight ... '

******

It is well documented that obesity is a social construction. This is true in both a more and a less obvious sense. The average weight has increased in developed societies because of increased availability of food and decreased exercise. At the same time, the meanings and values attached to body size and shape have also changed, with time and culture. In the West and in many other societies, fat bodies used to be regarded as aesthetically pleasing and sexually desirable.[10] In the early twentieth century, for example, the slender woman was regarded—in the words of a contemporary text—as the 'type of women men should shun when choosing a life companion'.[11] Such women, the writers went on,

> were 'man haters'. Their sexual development is arrested in early youth, as evidenced by 'flat chests, narrow hips, bloodless and thin or peaked features ... and a lack of that warmth and softness that attracts and holds the affections of men'.[12]

Many cultures have regarded fat as a desirable and aesthetically pleasing characteristic. Fatness is often a mark of social status for men and of marriageability in women. Large bodies are seen as soft and well tended by a prosperous, caring community.[13] They are also seen as sexually responsive and desirable. Rebecca Popenoe has shown how, for example, the 'laboriously fattened, voluptuous, immobile' bodies of Azawagh Arab women embody ideals of sexual desire, kinship, religion and health.[14] The women control the fattening process and with it establish their own social and sexual power. In Azawagh society, the beauty ideals attached to fatness are actively embraced by both sexes as an effective means of preserving the identity and solidarity of the community and the wellbeing of the individuals within it.

Fatness, therefore, may be a signifier of beauty and health, opulence and prosperity, power, sexual availability, dependent and domestic femininity and community wellbeing.[15] Obesity, on the other hand, is none of these things. It is not widely recognised that the concept—and indeed the word itself—is of relatively recent origin. The word 'obese' first appeared in English in the seventeenth century, as opposed to the word 'fat', which goes back at least a thousand years earlier. Obesity is a form of fatness that is linked to a series of moral and cultural valuations. It refers to excess and has progressively become linked to disease and other socially undesirable characteristics. Over time, the word has accumulated a congeries of connotations, which now include social transgression, greed, psychological maladjustment, impoverishment, untrustworthiness, self-indulgence and hedonism.[16] Studies have shown that physicians describe their obese patients as weak-willed, ugly and awkward.[17] Furthermore, as Jo has found many times, social discrimination against obese people is active and widespread.

Because obesity is a social construct, it is not surprising that, as in previous health issues configured at the cultural level as epidemics or plagues[18], it has been used in the service of larger social, economic and political projects. Bodies' surfaces and boundaries are continually crafted within social fields of inequality.[19] The feminist author Susan Bordo has argued that flesh gendered feminine is devalued in the pursuit of productive individualism and virtuous self-mastery.[20]

Katherine Le Besco has shown how meanings surrounding identities are produced on the basis of body size, which in turn produces social stigma.[21] 'Negotiating questions of fat identity', she writes, 'involves a fluid, alternating pattern of invocation and refusal of mainstream tropes of health, nature, and beauty'.[22]

> [C]urrent discourse surrounding body size and shape has worked to incorporate the protests of fat people against their own bodies; when civil rights are being demanded on the basis of genetic subjection of fat people, the fat body is effectively rendered uninhabitable.[23]

It is important to emphasise, however, that the various meanings of fatness are not just of purely theoretical interest, a curiosity of linguistic usage. These meanings are actually realised in the social flesh: they are engraved in bodies, which carry the traces of evolving traditions, fashions and aesthetic styles, and they result in real pain, real suffering and, too often, real despair.

Jo is not just a mind in a body, as in a box, and a body in the world. Her world itself is flesh. Her body is not 'in' the world and the world is not 'in' her body, ultimately. The world neither surrounds her flesh nor is surrounded by it. There is reciprocal insertion and intertwining of one in the other.[24]

Jo's body is at once an organon of knowledge and the source of the valuation of things. As Merleau-Ponty has said:

> There is a strict ideality in experiences that are experiences of the flesh: the moments of the sonata, the fragments of the luminous field, adhere to one another with a cohesion without concept, which is of the same type as the cohesions of the parts of my body, or the cohesion of my body with the world. Is my body a thing, is it an idea? It is neither, being the measurant of all things.[25]

Contrary to the assumptions of contemporary medical discourse, the body is not a machine and is not subject to machine-like causality. There is no simple causal route by which the social forces are played out within people's bodies. The pathway from society to the inner schema of the body, from history to flesh, from culture to the lifeworld, is tortuous and complex.

Let us return again to Jo.

******

Jo could not remember a time when she was happy. She had always felt she was the black sheep of the family. She was somehow different—more sensitive, less interested in sport. She liked music and would spend hours by herself as a young teenager. She was always lonely. More than her sister, she was disturbed by her parents' problems and can recall the shame she felt when a school friend visited and witnessed a violent argument in which her mother threatened her father with a knife.

She longed to be like the other girls and to be regarded as attractive to the boys. Sometimes her friends tried to help her, but on one occasion this turned to disaster. When she was sixteen she went out on a blind date with a boy who was four years older than her. He took her to a pub, got her drunk and then took her home and raped her. Confused and ashamed, feeling sullied and defiled, she confided in no-one. She became more of a recluse, her only source of physical pleasure being food.

Soon after, she left school. She had never been very good at studying and the constant humiliation made each day a painful experience. Her parents were too involved in their own problems to care much. She took up an apprenticeship at a horse stable and lived alone in a hut at the back of the stables. She was the only girl and the other apprentices, failing to make headway with her sexually, continued the pattern of ridicule and humiliation, often hitting her over the head in a gesture of contempt.

This was a period she remembered as one of absolute desolation. The only mitigation was the kindness she experienced from her boss and his family. The boss's wife was the first to suggest a diet. At her suggestion, Jo visited a doctor and was given instructions about what she could and couldn't eat.

She described how much she wanted to lose weight, how much she just wanted to be normal. When the doctor told her what to do, it seemed so easy. But in reality it wasn't easy at all. Her dependence on food was too strong. Despite her best efforts, she couldn't resist the hunger. During the day she would try not to think of food by trying to focus on her work. During the night she would lie awake, sad and alone, trying to ignore the vast chasm in her stomach aching for the comfort of food, any food. Her whole body seemed to shout at her, command, compel her, to eat.

It would often reach the point where she could think of nothing else. She would turn on the television, try to think of things she would like to do, places she would like to visit, but it was often of no use. Sometimes she would go for a whole day, or nearly a day, eating almost nothing. She would get to ten o'clock at night and think to herself that she had made it: one day, one small accomplishment, perhaps a few grams less in weight. That, at least, would be an achievement of sorts. There was not much else to be proud of.

Sometimes she would get to ten o'clock and feel so bereft, so lonely, so sad, that without knowing how or why she would find herself at the local Seven-Eleven shop, buying a couple of pies and two cans of Coke. She would devour them, like a junkie taking a hit. The comfort was instantaneous but only momentary. Afterwards, she would inevitably feel more humiliated than ever, totally abject, defiled and negated, absolutely nothing.

******

How does a society enter a body? How does it shape our flesh? In the lifeworld, the intimate domain of immediate experience, sensuous and social, how are the structures of our bodily experiences and meanings composed and then given corporeal reality? Perhaps the most primordial of lifeworld experiences is that of the enjoyment of food. In spite of the fact that in modern medical and cultural discourses, eating is presented as a purely functional and physiological activity, from earliest memories it evokes rich and diverse significations. One does not have to invoke the ritual of fasting practised in virtually all cultures and all the major religious traditions, or the use of the hunger strike as a political weapon by Mahatma Gandhi, Bobby Sands, Daniel Berrigan, the suffragettes and many others as proof of this. One only has to reflect on the mundane act of eating itself.

The most powerful way in which cultural and social influences are imprinted on the body is through the experience of eating. Medical discourse has focused on the physiology of energy metabolism and hunger, and modern social and public health campaigns have sought to change eating attitudes and behaviour. However, eating is not a purely mechanical activity that can be modified at will according to dictates issued by doctors or policies promulgated by public health practitioners. The meanings of eating, and the habits and practices associated with it, evoke some of the most elemental and primal experiences of an individual and are closely bound up with their senses of personal and psychic identity. To understand these meanings, it is necessary to examine in detail what is involved. Let us reflect, therefore, on the mundane process of eating.

Here I am at breakfast. I am hungry. I know that I am hungry, because I am separated from the world. I am separate and needy, because I am human. I can see that the world stretching out before me exists to satiate my hunger.

I experience the anticipation of the meal. My attention focuses and my senses grow more acute as I respond to the sight and smell of the food: the toast, the egg, the orange juice. I arrange the food on the plate and adjust my position in my chair. I exclude other sensations. I place a morsel of the egg and toast in my mouth. The taste wells up, spreads through my mouth, suffuses my body. I feel slight contractions in my pharynx and upper abdomen. I savour the experience, try to hold the moment. I experience with pleasure the various textures, the crunching sensation, the mixture of flavours.

During enjoyment, as Emmanuel Levinas says, I am a hungry stomach without ears. I concentrate on my own pleasure. While I am savouring this mouthful of food, there is no physical distance between me and the world. I become my sensations. 'The objects of the world, which for thought lie in the void, for sensibility—or for life—spread forth on a horizon which entirely hides that void.'[26] This sensibility is my experience of otherness, of 'the elemental'.

In the satisfaction of need, the alienness of the world that founds me loses its alterity: in satiety, the real I sank my teeth into is assimilated, the forces that were in the other become my forces, become me (and every satisfaction of need is in some respect nourishment).[27]

I repeat my actions. I am now chewing methodically. I swallow and trace the passage of the macerated food into my upper pharynx and then I lose it, to discover a sense of fullness in my stomach. I establish a comforting rhythm, involving my jaw, my tongue, my hands and my throat. I repeat the actions without thinking—in fact, it takes some effort to stop. The rhythm is reassuring, calming. The external environment has receded from my consciousness. My whole body is focused on the gustatory experience. I am embraced by it, consumed by the act of consuming.

In enjoyment, to quote Levinas again, I am absolutely for myself. I am alone without solitude, innocently egoist and alone. Not against the Other, not 'as for me', but entirely deaf to the Other, outside all communication and all refusal to communicate.[28]

> The signification of the gustatory and the olfactory, of eating and enjoying, has to be sought on the basis of the signifyingness of signification, the one for the other ... It is a passivity more passive still than any passivity that is antithetical to an act, a nudity more naked than all 'academic' nudity, exposed to the point of outpouring, effusion and prayer. It is a passivity that is not reducible to exposure to another's gaze. It is a vulnerability and a paining exhausting themselves like a haemorrhage ... [29]

After a time I am aware of a fullness in my stomach, but the plate still beckons. The hand-to-mouth actions continue without my conscious intervention. The sense of pleasant fullness may be exceeded. Even if I am not really concerned about my weight, I connect the act of eating with a sense of weightiness. Each mouthful connotes a sense of excess. I have a mental image of obese persons; not myself, but others. The disapproval associated with eating—overeating—surrounds me. I feel a mixture of guilt, pleasure, excess, self-betrayal. I am suffused with a variety of sensations, not all of them consistent: pleasant satisfaction, comfort, reassurance, shame.

When I am in the process of satiating my hunger, my relationship with the world changes. When I eat, I am not distant from the world: I am absorbed in it. I am overwhelmed with it sensually. I taste it and feel it and enjoy the developing sensation of satiation. This is my absorption in the element, and my first experience of the world's otherness.[30]

******

Jo and I have reflected many times on the question, What is the space one seeks to fill by eating? One thing is clear: it is rarely, if ever, a physiological space. Rather, it is a space of meaning and values. It is a space to be filled by a caring, nurturing relationship with the world and with others. It is a space to be filled by solidity, comfort, gentleness and reassurance.

The 'body naked and indigent identifies the centre of the world it perceives', says Levinas. It conditions it by its own representations of the world 'and is thereby torn from the centre from which it proceeded, as water gushing forth from rock washes away that rock'. The body indigent and naked is not a thing among things. It is 'the very reverting ... of representation into life, of the subjectivity that represents into life which is sustained by these representations and lives off them'.[31] The world I constitute nourishes me and bathes me. It is aliment and 'medium'.[32]

Eating is an activity of meaning that is both intensely personal and deeply social. In fact, there is a surplus of meaning. Representation consists in the possibility of accounting for the object as though it were constituted by a thought, but there is an overflowing of meaning that arises in relation to alimentation. The surplus over meaning is not a meaning in its turn, simply thought as a condition—which would be to reduce the aliment to a correlate represented.

> Eating ... is not reducible ... to the set of gustative, olfactory, kinaesthetic, and other sensations that would constitute the consciousness of eating. This sinking one's teeth into the things which the act of eating involves above all measures the surplus of the reality of the aliment over every represented reality, a surplus that is not quantitative, but is the way the I, the absolute commencement, is suspended on the non-I. The corporeity of the living being and its indigence as a naked and hungry body is the accomplishment of these structures ... [33]

The eating process is a sensual one and, indeed, the model for all enjoyment and satisfaction. However, something can go wrong in the moment of pure sensibility.[34] Instead of the element serving as an access to satiation and pleasure, it can deliver me abstractly over to otherness, into pure empty sensibility.[35] Faceless and losing itself in nothingness, my body can become inscribed in the fathomless depth of the elements.[36] Darkness is the very play of existence that would play itself out even if there were nothing. There is a density, an atmosphere, a field in which I become immersed, which omits the actual objects that would have this density, which lies outside the breath of existence or the field of familiar forces.[37]

Jo was all too familiar with both the ecstasy and the agony of eating. For her, eating was a source of solace. Her layers of fat provided insulation against the assaults of the inexorable harshness of the world. Her expanding body was her panoply, her shield. It protected her, but, paradoxically, it also exposed her. Not only was it a shield to hide behind, it also stripped her bare. It rendered her completely naked, exposed to anyone who merely glanced at her, who could in an instant read her inner fears, her passions, her weaknesses and her pain.

As with other major illnesses throughout history, the obese body is a nodal point for conflicting lines of force: for negative surges, humiliation, disease metaphors, decay and abandon, resistance, opposition. It is a palimpsest for diverse meanings, the site of cultural inscriptions that are not always clearly legible and not always consistent. It is a kind of cultural lightning rod—a focus of fear and fantasises, aspirations and ambitions. It may be regarded as the site of plenitude, or luxury, or wealth or power; that is, it may be at the heart of the social order and its institutions. It may also be the site of excess, of the absence of control, of abandon, of unrestrained libido. The obese body may therefore be marginalised, outcast, darkly threatening—the imminent breakdown of internal and external control.

******

Jo never finished the apprenticeship. After a couple of years she left the stables and drifted a bit. She worked in various jobs and had a couple of unsuccessful relationships from which she ended up with two children. She tried alcohol and speed, but they didn't do much for her. She thought a lot about death and wondered about killing herself, but she never tried anything.

When she was thirty-eight she teamed up with Damien, who was ten years younger and himself had problems with depression and drugs. However, he truly cared for her and committed himself to the care of her children, who were now teenagers. He suggested that she seek specialist help and, on her GP's advice, she came to see me.

By this time her medical problems were far advanced and she had great difficulty breathing as well as walking. But what upset and humiliated her most was her inability to care for herself at the most mundane level. She needed help from Damien or one of the children to dress, wash or even clean herself after going to the toilet. In addition to her deep personal demoralisation, she now also felt that she was failing her family. It had been one thing to have betrayed herself; she now felt that she was also betraying the only truly caring relationship she had ever experienced.

She was desperate to seek a solution. We discussed surgery. The image of the surgeon's knife slashing at her skin was almost unbearable, but she suppressed her revulsion and spoke with a surgeon, only to find that there would be no way she and Damien could afford the thousands of dollars needed to proceed.

******

Jo had over many years grown to hate her body. She was not alone. For everyone else, it also seemed to be an object of abhorrence and disgust. She was, in fact, often taken aback by the intensity of the attacks on her, as she was merely going about her daily business. It was as if they thought that *she* was attacking *them*, as if she posed a threat against which they had to defend themselves. She could not understand how, raw and vulnerable as she was—her only defence, her pathetic and ineffectual defence, being her thick layers of adipose tissue—how *she* could be encountered as menacing, as a figure of abhorrence and dread.

The obese body—like all bodies—is not just one body but many. It is the biological body, the body of organs and tissues, of health, sickness and disease. It is also the social and cultural body, the body of affect and emotions, the body of love and hate, of imagination and dreams, of hope and dread, of guilt, of sin, of sexuality and passion, of scandalous transgressions, of dark secrets and unspoken desires. It is the body of forces and densities, of drives and inner, unknown spaces.[38]

The body of medicine is one of the proudest achievements of reason and the Enlightenment. In this canon, the body is made up of spaces and volumes. It is presented as entirely finished, completed, strictly limited, and is shown from the outside as something individual. That which transgresses its limits is excluded, hidden or moderated, including sexual life, eating, drinking and defecation, which are transferred to the private and psychological levels where their connotations become narrow and specific, torn away from a direct relation to the life of society and to the cosmic whole.[39] It is self-sufficient and speaks in its name alone. In the medical discourse, death is only death and never coincides with birth; old age is torn away from youth. All actions and events are interpreted on the level of a single, individual life. They are enclosed within the limits of the same body, limits that are the absolute beginning and end and can never meet.[40]

The body of science is the full, multifarious body attenuated and purified of all its inconvenient and carnal excrescences. The elements that reason sought so assiduously to subdue, however, could not be extirpated altogether. Instead, they were forced underground, into more arcane social and psychological locations, from which they continued to wage an obdurate war of resistance. Historically, one of the manifestations of these recondite remnants of pre-Enlightenment reason was the figure of the grotesque body, which erupted from time to time in carnivals and other events when social discipline was momentary loosened.[41] The obese body is one of the contemporary forms of this arcane space.

The grotesque body provided all the elements that were lost when the rational, medical body was constructed: the merging of life and death, the continuity with the ancestral body, which is renewed in the next generation, and with other fleshly bodies. It was a body in the act of becoming, never finished, never completed, continually built and created, and subject to unlimited transformation. It swallowed the world and was itself swallowed by the world. It ignored the impenetrable surface that closed and limited bodies as separate and completed phenomena.

In the contemporary age, the bulges and eruptions, the rolls of fat, the uncontainable surfaces and volumes of the obese body, suggests 'uncontained desire, unrestrained hunger, uncontrolled impulses', a refusal of regimentation and subjection.[42] In this sense, the obese body is a body opposed to science, standing against science, and by its nature resisting the epistemological and social discipline imposed by scientific thought and the practices that accompany it.

As a component of the grotesque, the obese body offers a gesture of resistance to the totalising sway of science and medicine. But, as every obese person knows, this is not a war of liberation. In the contemporary world, the other of science and knowledge is experienced, not as pleasure and creative enjoyment, but as shame and revulsion, as disgust and horror, as abjection.

Abjection and the grotesque are two sides of one coin. They reflect the same characteristics of the obese body: its ambiguity, and the fact that it does not respect borders, positions and rules. As abjection, the obese body disturbs identity, system and order. It is a place not where meaning is created but where it collapses, where 'I' am not.[43] The abject, obese body presents a life-threatening negation that must be radically excluded. The abject is the in-between, what defies boundaries, a composite resistant to unity, the threat of unassimilable non-unity.[44]

The experience of abjection is frequently described not only by those observing obese bodies but by the obese people themselves. The following description by Julia Kristeva evokes Jo's poignant descriptions of her own corporeal experience:

> [There is] a weight of meaningless, about which there is nothing insignificant, and which crushes me ... [45] There looms ... one of those violent, dark revolts of being, directed against a threat that seems to emanate from an exorbitant, outside or inside, ejected beyond the scope of the possible, the tolerable, the thinkable. It lies there, quite close, but it cannot be assimilated. It beseeches, worries, and fascinates desire, which, nevertheless, does not let itself be seduced.[46]

In the classical account of Mary Douglas, filth and defilement exist on the border of identities and threaten the unity of the ego. Revulsion and disgust are referents to those things that cannot be controlled, which refuse to be bounded and are anomalies that cause profound cultural anxiety. The rolls of fat, the flab, the surfeit of tissue, the seepages and discharges, all signify the disorder that threatens whenever the injunction to consume is taken too literally and the precarious balance of psychic and social discipline breaks down.[47] The boundaries between the pure and the dangerous are largely conventional: today, the obese body stands on the side of danger.

Abjection is, therefore, systematically generated deep within the culture. There is an inescapable need for objects of revilement. They help maintain social solidarity and guarantee psychological coherence. Like other plagues before it, obesity exquisitely epitomises the fears and terror deep within the contemporary social imaginary. In the public sphere of contemporary society, fat bodies have assumed the function of the abject: as 'that which must be expelled to make all other bodily representations and functions, even life itself, possible'.[48] They take up the burden of representing the horror of the body itself for the culture at large. They symbolise the inevitable death and decay of all bodies, the inexorable fate of all carnal matter.

******

Jo's body bore the stigmata of her sad life. There is a cruel and ironic parallel between her body, the merciless reception of it, the medical consequences and the facts of her social and emotional life.

Jo was by now unable to undertake even the most meagre of physical actions. When surgery had been excluded, all that was left was the strategy that had failed her all her life: resisting the compulsion to eat. It was futile, and we both knew it, but she promised to try it all the same. On one occasion over three months, her weight fell by 5 kg. We tried to maintain a façade of hopefulness. The next time, however, her weight had gone up again.

She was increasingly remorseful and full of self-blame. She had tried to break out of the circle of hopelessness. But the forces against her had been too powerful. She knew she was beaten, or at least that she couldn't win. She asked about the effects of stopping her medications. I explained what the role of each one was. She assured me that she was not suicidal and would not attempt to take her own life.

She knew that she was caught in a trap, that the wound in her flesh was deep and immedicable. She was an innocent bystander to her own tragedy.

I last saw Jo just before Christmas. She was happier than usual and talked optimistically about the forthcoming family celebrations. But she failed to attend her next appointment a month later. Her husband rang later that day to say that, tragically, he had found her dead beside him in their bed that morning. It appeared that she had died of natural causes.

******

The obesity epidemic is not merely a crisis of health outcomes or health care costs. It is a symptom of deeper processes within medicine and the culture. The obese body is not just a body of health, sickness and disease. It is many bodies, including the bodies of society and culture, the emotions, imagination, sin and sexuality. It is a space of excess, of surplus of meaning, of resistance against the relentless, unpitying forces of the apparatuses of science and culture. It is also a site of sadness, of humiliation, of loss, of abject defeat.

Our bodies are not just objects in the world. We are, to be sure, flesh and blood, atoms and molecules, hormones and electrical impulses. But we are also flows, movements, strata, segments, intensities, aligned and linked in heterogeneous, disparate, discontinuous unities.[49]

This has been the story of one body, a body that was ravaged, abused and, until the end, uncared for. This essay is dedicated to Jo herself and all those who suffered with her.

Notes

1. Lord Byron, 'Childe Harold's Pilgrimage: Canto the Fourth', in McGann, ed., *Byron: The Complete Poetical Works* (Oxford, Clarendon Press, The Oxford English Texts series, 1980–93).
2. M Merleau-Ponty, *Phenomenology of Perception* (London, Routledge and Kegan Paul, 1962), p. 70.
3. E Husserl, *Cartesian Meditations: An Introduction to Phenomenology*, tr. D Cairns (The Hague, Martinus Nijhoff, 1960), pp. 116–17; E Husserl, *Ideas Pertaining to a Pure Phenomenology and to a Phenomenological Philosophy: Studies in the Phenomenology of Constitution*, trs Rojcewicz and A Schuwer (Dordrecht, Kluwer Academic Publishers, 1989), pp. 165–6; A Schutz and T Luckmann, *The Structures of the Life-world*, trs Richard M Zaner and H Tristram Engelhardt (London, Heinemann, 1974), pp. 222–6.
4. E Grosz, *Volatile Bodies* (Bloomington, Indiana University Press, 1994), p. 102.
5. RM Zaner, *Conversations on the Edge: Narratives of Ethics and Illness*

(Washington, DC, Georgetown University Press, 2004); RM Zaner, *Ethics and the Clinical Encounter* (Edgeworth Cliffs, NJ, Prentice-Hall, 1988).
6   For example, E Grosz, *Volatile Bodies*, and J Butler, *Gender Trouble: Feminism and the Subversion of Identity* (New York, Routledge, 1990).
7   For example, SK Toombs, *The Meaning of Illness: A Phenomenological Account of the Different Perspectives of Physician and Patient* (Dordrecht and Boston, Kluwer Academic Publishers, 1992).
8   SK Toombs, 'The Lived Experience of Disability', *Human Studies*, 18, 1995: 9–23.
9   cf. S Murray, '(Un/Be)Coming Out? Rethinking Fat Politics', *Social Semiotics*, 15(2), 2005: 153–63.
10 A Jutel, 'Weighing Health: The Moral Burden of Obesity', *Social Semiotics*, 15(2), 2005: 113–25.
11 GP Wood and EH Rudduck, *Vitalogy or Encyclopedia of House and Home* (Chicago, Vitalogy Association, 1923), quoted in A Jutel, 'Weighing Health'.
12 ibid., p. 861, quoted in A Jutel, 'Weighing Health'.
13 M Mauss, *The Gift: Forms and Functions of Exchange in Archaic Societies*, tr. Ian Cunnison (New York, Norton, 1967).
14 R Popenoe, *Feeding Desire: Fatness, Beauty, and Sexuality among a Saharan People* (London, Routledge, 2004).
15 H Gremillion, 'The Cultural Politics of Body Size, Annu. Rev., *Anthropol*, 34, 2005: 13–32; see also A Jutel, 'Weighing Health'.
16 J Polivy, D Garner and P Garfinkel, 'Causes and Consequences of the Current Preference for Thin Female Physiques', in CP Herman, MP Zanna and ET Higgins, eds, *Physical Appearance, Stigma and Social Behavior* (Hillsdale, NJ, Lawrence Erlbaum, 1986).
17 GL Maddox and V Liederman, 'Overweight as a Social Disability with Medical Implications', *Journal of Medical Education*, 44, 1969: 214–20.
18 S Sontag, *Illness as Metaphor* (London, Penguin, 1991).
19 J Butler, *Gender Trouble*, and J Butler, *Bodies that Matter: On the Discursive Limits of 'Sex'* (New York, 1993, Routledge).
20 S Bordo, *Unbearable Weight* (Berkeley, University of California Press, 1993), p. 142.
21 JE Braziel and K Le Besco, eds, *Bodies out of Bounds: Fatness and Transgression* (Berkeley, University of California Press, 2001).
22 A Losano and BA Risch, 'Resisting Venus: Negotiating Corpulence in Exercise Videos', in JE Braziel and K Le Besco, eds, *Bodies out of Bounds*, p. 123. The most obvious of these is the medical one. In the medical interpretation obesity relates to dietary management. According to Bryan Turner this 'emerged out of a theology of the flesh, developed through a moralistic medicine and finally established itself as a science of the efficient body'; see B Turner, *The Body and Society: Explorations in Social Theory* (London, Sage, 1984), p. 3.
23 K Le Besco, 'Queering Fat Bodies/politics', in JE Braziel and K Le Besco, eds, *Bodies out of Bounds*, p. 76.
24 M Merleau-Ponty, *The Visible and the Invisible*, ed. Claude Lefort, tr. Alphonso Lingis (Evanston, North-western University Press, 1968), p. 138.

25 ibid., p 152.
26 E Levinas, *Totality and Infinity*, tr. Alphonso Lingis (Hingham, MA, M. Nijhoff, 1979), p. 135.
27 ibid., p. 128.
28 ibid., p. 134.
29 ibid., p. 127.
30 E Levinas, *Otherwise than Being*, tr. Alphonso Lingis (Hingham, MA, M. Nijhoff, 1979), p. 72.
31 E Levinas, *Totality and Infinity*, p. 127.
32 ibid., p. 128.
33 ibid., p. 128.
34 E Levinas, *Existence and Existents*, tr. Alphonso Lingis (The Hague, M. Nijhoff, 1978), pp. 56–8.
35 ibid., p. 57.
36 E Levinas, *Totality and Infinity*, p. 158.
37 E Levinas, 'There Is: Existence without Existents', in S Hand, ed., *The Levinas Reader* (London, Blackwell, 2001), p. 35.
38 G Deleuze and F Guattari, *A Thousand Plateaus: Capitalism and Schizophrenia*, tr. Brian Massumi (Minneapolis, University of Minnesota Press, 1987), p. 30.
39 MM Bakhtin, *Rabelais and His World*, tr. Helene Iswolsky (Cambridge, MA, MIT Press, 1968).
40 ibid.
41 ibid.
42 S Bordo, *Unbearable Weight*, p. 189.
43 Julia Kristeva, *Powers of Horror: An Essay on Abjection*, tr. Leon S Roudiez (New York, Columbia University Press, 1982), p. 26.
44 See J Lechte, *Julia Kristeva* (London and New York, Routledge, 1990), pp. 157–67.
45 Julia Kristeva, *Powers of Horror*, p. 2.
46 ibid., p. 1.
47 M Douglas, *Purity and Danger: An Analysis of Concepts of Pollution and Taboo* (London, Routledge, 2002 [1966]), p. 2.
48 L Kent, 'Fighting Abjection', in JE Braziel and K Le Besco, eds, *Bodies out of Bounds*, p. 135.
49 G Deleuze and F Guattari, *A Thousand Plateaus*, p. 152.

Chapter 13
The Case of Miss T

The following is an edited transcript of a discussion at a conference on the theory and practice of ethics in medicine. The participants included doctors, nurses, social workers, philosophers and laypeople with an interest in ethics.

> PK: I'd like to tell you about the case of an elderly woman I once looked after and to ask your opinions about what I should have done at the time. It was a difficult and complex case, which made a big impact on me—indeed, even today, years later, scarcely a day goes by without some aspect of it recurring to me in one way or another.
>
> I was working as a medical registrar at a large public hospital at the time. The patient, whom I eventually came to know very well, had already been seen over many years at the hospital. She was regarded as something of a medical curiosity because she had a collection of odd conditions, thought to be 'autoimmune' in character—that means that the body turns on itself and attacks its own tissues. When I first met her she was seventy-eight years old. She'd had a long history of rheumatoid arthritis, which although it was no longer active or caused her pain had left her body

ravaged and debilitated. She also had chronic liver and lung conditions, and it was this last one which caused her the most problems. It made her breathless—so much so that for years she'd been unable to walk more than a few steps at a time—and it affected her heart, so that she retained fluid in her legs and her lungs.

She took a large number of medications, which for a considerable period had served her very well. In spite of the physical limitations she remained mentally active and alert, and indeed, managed to tend the garden in her small house, of which she was very proud. I visited her house once—using some excuse, because I'd heard her talk so much about it and was curious. She'd lived there for nearly forty years, and it was her whole world, which she'd fashioned lovingly and with great care and subtlety. The garden too was a source of joy to her, and she proudly showed me around her rose garden and her vegetable patch.

Miss T had never married and had lived almost all her life alone. Evidently, she'd been somewhat of a rebel in her day—certainly, a 'modern woman'. She'd decided early that she'd have an independent career, and she went to university where she gained a degree in English. She later became a teacher and eventually was a respected English mistress at a private school for girls. Literature was her life and love, and she could speak for hours about books she'd read and places she'd visited in her imagination.

As I said, she never married. I understand that she'd had a number of relationships and that her liberated lifestyle had in its day raised a few eyebrows. But she never compromised her independence. She bought her own house and supported herself, even in the face of her considerable medical problems.

I didn't ever find out much about her family. In fact, the only family I came to know about was an elderly sister, with whom she remained close all her life, and a niece. The sister, who was eighty-two, herself suffered from osteoarthritis of the hips, which together with her considerable obesity, substantially limited her mobility. She lived a few kilometres away. The niece was in her late twenties or early thirties and, I think, was still a student. She'd developed quite a close attachment to her aunt and visited her every week or so and helped with shopping and cleaning. Incidentally, I should mention that for years Miss T had received the maximum available community supports, including council help, Meals on Wheels, visiting nurses when required and so on.

The story I want to discuss with you in fact started some time before I knew her. Miss T had been going to a general practitioner for many years—he was almost as old as she was. They'd come to know each other reasonably well and would often chat about current affairs and books they were reading. As I understand it, on a number of occasions she'd raised with him the possibility of her becoming so disabled that she'd no longer be able to care for herself. She stated directly and unequivocally many times that if she were to lose her independence she wouldn't want to go on living. She'd said to the doctor that if she could no longer follow the style of life of her choice, she'd want him to give her something to help her die.

Well, it so happens that her condition gradually deteriorated, to the point where it was apparent to the GP that she could no longer reasonably manage at home on her own. Furthermore, given the inexorable nature of her condition, it was clear to him that in due course she'd require quite substantial nursing support. Accordingly, he told her that he thought that the time had come where she had seriously to consider entering a nursing home. Miss T replied something like: 'We've discussed many times how my independence is most precious to me. I don't want to go on living in circumstances in which my lifestyle is not of my choosing. Please give me something to make me die'.

I'd like you to imagine that you were the local doctor. What would you do? What should he have done? Before answering this, perhaps if anyone has some factual questions they would like clarified, we should do that first.

A: I have two small questions. First, what sort of medications was she taking?

PK: She was taking some medications for her heart failure—digoxin and a diuretic, if I remember correctly—and inhaled Ventolin for her asthma. I think that was all.

A: And how disabled was she from all her conditions at this time? I mean, could she walk, use her hands and so on?

PK: This was a bit before I knew her, and I can really only speak about the later time in detail. But as I understand it, at that point she really couldn't walk more than a few steps at a time without getting short of breath. Her hands were distorted and she'd had to have special taps put into the house and that sort of thing, but that was a chronic problem which I don't think had changed much for some years.
If you were the GP, what would you do in his position?

B: It's hard to answer without being there, but if it's her wish to die—and it seems that she's thought it out carefully and it's not just a spur-of-the-moment thing—then she should be able to do as she pleases. I mean, she's an autonomous person, isn't she, and she has the right to decide whether she'll live and die.

C: But she's actually asking the GP to help her and that's another thing. If I was her GP I think I'd find it very hard to help her, especially after knowing her all those years.

D: I don't think that she has the right to ask the doctor to kill her. Anyway, that's not his job. She's asking him to do something that has nothing to do with doctoring.

B: I disagree with that. The doctor's job is to relieve suffering, and this woman is suffering. Helping her die would just be a continuation of what he'd been trying to do all along.

E: No. The doctor's job is to preserve life, not to take it. To kill her would be to betray everything that medicine stands for. Anyway, if she really wanted to die, she could do it herself—she could just go away and take poison, or something.

F: But she mightn't know how to do it. A lot of people don't—including me! Anyway, if she tried and failed, it could be very distressing.

PK: I think some of that is true. When I knew her, she'd often say that her independence and her books and so on were very important to her but that she never wanted to suffer. 'I've never liked pain', she once said to me, ironically, 'yet I've had so much of it'.

B: D, don't you think that it should be her choice whether she lives or dies? She's a mature adult. Why shouldn't she make up her own mind?

D: It is not that she shouldn't make up her own mind; it's that she's imposing on the doctor to kill her. I think that's wrong.

G: *(With intensity)* I think it's the other way round: it's the doctor who's on the power trip. I really can't see what the point of this is …

F: Perhaps the doctor doesn't actually have to kill her but could tell her what to do, how to do it quickly and painlessly …

B: Perhaps he could give her a normal prescription of pills and tell her that if she took all of them at once it would kill her.

F: That's a bit like the suicide machine we were talking about earlier today, isn't it? It would then be her decision and she'd be carrying it out.

E: I'm very surprised by the way this discussion is going! Everyone has assumed that because she's said that she wants to die once that's all there is to it …

B: She's said it on many occasions …

E: People say all sorts of things when they are sick or distressed. She's probably upset that he's told her that she has to go and live in a nursing home. I know I would be. It's natural for her to think about ending it all. But she might change. She might get to like it. She hasn't even tried it out.

PK: So, E, what would you do if you were in the situation of the GP?

E: Well, I'm not a doctor, but I suppose you'd have to talk with her and make her understand that it's not the end of the world, but that she's just entering a new phase of her life. It may even turn out to be very satisfying for her. In particular, it might bring her closer to God, if she's religious.

B: (*Becoming heated*) Look, I think that that's just incredibly paternalistic! She's made up her mind and we have to respect that.

PK: What would you do, B?

B: I wouldn't kill her outright because I don't want to go to jail, though if I could do it legally I would. I don't think there's any difference between giving someone pills to kill themselves and giving them an injection, except that the injection would probably work better! In the circumstances, I'd probably give her some tablets or tell her what tablets to take or something like that, like F suggested. But I think she's got a right to die if she wants to.

(*Calls of 'No!' and 'You can't kill her!'*)

PK: Unless I'm wrong, B and F are in the minority. Although a number of you are in sympathy with her wish to die, no-one else would take active steps either to kill her or to facilitate her death. Is that right? Well, it so happens that the GP refused to help her die. I suppose you already guessed that: if he hadn't, there wouldn't have been a story for me to tell.

The GP refused and she went home. A few days after this she was admitted to hospital, and this was when I met Miss T for the first time. She had an exacerbation of her lung and heart conditions. When I first saw her, she was certainly in a bad way. She had severe oedema—that is, fluid retention—extending from her feet right up to her waist. She was so short of breath that she literally couldn't sit up without gasping for air, and she was certainly unable to stand up or walk. All this was superimposed on her tiny, emaciated body with its distortions from chronic rheumatoid arthritis.

During her stay in hospital, which lasted about four weeks, I came to know her quite well. In spite of her debility, she was an engaging and lively woman who loved to talk about life and people. She gave me an account of her earlier life—her determination to live the way she wanted and not to conform to the stereotypes of the times, not to marry or to become a housewife. She was proud of her achievements too. As I said before, she loved her home and her books, and was never happier than when talking about some work of literature that an event or circumstance had reminded her of, or quoting an apt verse of poetry. She painted a vivid picture of her own life, and of what had driven her. 'I've drunk life to the lees', she used to say grandiosely. 'I've been happy and I've suffered too.'

I think I'm not being immodest to say that Miss T came to regard me as a kind of surrogate grandson—and the warmth was mutual.

D: Did she ever discuss with you her wish to die?

PK: No, not once. She never raised the question directly,

although she came close. She certainly said enough to have made it clear where her priorities lay and what was most important to her. I learnt about what had happened before she came into hospital from the GP. Although we never talked about it openly, I'm convinced that she knew that I was aware of her conversations with him on the subject of dying.

During her stay in hospital, with bed rest and diuretic therapy, her condition improved substantially and after a while she was able to move around a bit and to care for herself. We discussed her future and our feeling that she really needed to enter full-time care. After lengthy discussions she agreed to try a nursing home. Luckily, she had a bit of money, so it was possible to find a place for her in one of the better nursing homes.

She left the hospital on a Wednesday morning and was taken straight to the nursing home by taxi. We'd made elaborate arrangements for her sister and niece to go to her house and get whatever things she needed; she was going to try out the nursing home for a few weeks and, if she liked it, she'd eventually sell or rent out her house to pay the bills.

However, the very next morning, Thursday morning, I received a phone call from the Sister in Charge at the nursing home. Miss T had been at the place for less than twenty-four hours and, sick and debilitated as she was, she was out in the street hailing a taxi. I think that this gives a good indication of her personality and of her sheer strength of will. When I spoke to her some time later she explained that the nursing home was just as she'd expected: the food was terrible, the nurses and doctors condescended to her as if she was senile, and the other inhabitants were, as she put it, 'just a lot of old fogies sitting around waiting to die!'

The nursing home, it seems, wasn't for her. She caught the taxi not to her own home but to her sister's place. And there they stayed together for some months. I forget how long it was—maybe two or three months. I never visited them at home, but I have a vivid mental image of what must have happened: the two elderly women, each almost as debilitated as the other, one very obese and hardly able to get about herself, and the other terribly deformed and gasping for breath, grappling to get each other dressed or to the toilet. It must have been an amazing sight! It was also an indication of the spirit and mutual commitment of the two sisters.

Anyway, they managed like this for some months. During this time, Miss T continued to attend hospital outpatients on a regular basis. She'd be wheeled in in a wheelchair by her sister or a nurse and we'd discuss her medications. Her pride at having escaped the nursing home was evident.

A: Was she compliant with her medications?

PK: Yes, indeed. She was a model patient. Her medical condition was more or less stable for a time. Then one day, just at the end of the consultation, exactly as she was about to leave the consulting room, she said, 'Oh, Doctor, there's just one more thing …'

C: That means trouble …

PK: Yes, when you hear this at the end of a clinical consultation your heart usually sinks, especially if you're in a hurry, because you know that something important is about to emerge. In any case, as you can imagine, appointments with Miss T always took longer than those with other patients.

'Yes', I said.

'This morning, while washing, I noticed something in my breast. Would you mind having a look at it?'

I helped her on to the couch again and undressed her. I examined her breasts and found a lump in the right breast that seemed to me clinically very likely to be a cancer. What should I do?

B: Tell her, of course.

PK: Tell her what?

B: That you think it is a cancer. I can't see the problem.

PK: But I don't know yet that that is what it is. It is only my suspicion.

B: Then say that to her. Say that you need to do some tests to confirm it.

PK: Do I need to do tests? Would that make a difference?

B: Give her the option! Say something like 'I can't be absolutely sure yet, but I think that you might have a cancer. We need to do some tests to confirm it'.

F: She wanted to die not long ago. She now has a condition that could help her die. Why not just leave it?

E: But has she said that she wants to die? It seems to me that she's going pretty well at her sister's and that dying's no longer an issue.

A: But her condition's going to get worse soon. If she was that sick when she came into hospital it's only a matter of time. It might be better to bring the subject up with her again.

PK: But she hasn't said to me that she wants to die. Should I raise the issue with her? What do you suggest? Perhaps I could introduce the subject by saying something like 'Remember once you wanted to die … '?

G: Look, I think this discussion is a waste of time! Why don't we talk about something important? All you need to do is use your communication skills. I came here to discuss ethics, not the irrelevant and paternalistic things doctors who think they're God say to their clients!

PK: I'm sorry to offend you, G, but I think we *are* talking about ethics. We're talking about what you actually do in face-to-face situations that require decisions about issues of value. Can you tell us what you would say to Miss T?

G: You just talk to her and you tell her what the facts are. I can't see what the problem is.

PK: Perhaps we can pretend that I'm the patient at this point in the consultation. What are the exact words you'd use, G?

(Pause)

C: What did you say to her?

PK: Well, as far as I can remember, I said something like 'Yes, I can feel a lump and I am concerned about it. We could do some tests if you wish. What do you want me to do?' That seems ideologically sound, doesn't it?
    She said, 'What do you recommend?'
    In fact, she said this often. Although she was a strong, vivid and opinionated character—very opinionated!—she was always extremely meticulous about following any advice I'd give; sometimes, this was to the point where it was embarrassing to me. She'd say, 'Tell me what to do. You're the doctor. I know nothing about medicine; my field is English literature'. She thought this was rather a witty line and repeated it often.

A: That happens all the time. Patients always ask doctors to tell them what to do. They don't want a medical textbook; they want a prescription.

C: I agree with that. People come to doctors for advice and help about the things that doctors are good at. They trust them and do what they say.

E: But it's not as simple as that, as this very case shows. It's not just a matter of technical decision-making. The technical decisions can't be separated from the questions of life and death, the questions of a personal and maybe spiritual kind that the doctor has no business interfering in.

D: Could you give us who aren't familiar with this area a bit of information? What are the options here?

PK: A or C might be able to answer that better than I can, but under normal circumstances, I think, the procedure would be to confirm the diagnosis with some kind of biopsy procedure. If a carcinoma were proven in this age group it would normally be removed. Often a removal of the lump would be enough, although sometimes the whole breast is still removed. The woman would then have some additional therapy—X-ray therapy perhaps, and then maybe some hormone treatment.

A: She'd be a very bad anaesthetic risk. An operation would probably kill her.

PK: That's a reasonable point, but perhaps a lumpectomy could be done with regional anaesthesia.

D: What would happen if you did nothing?

PK: There are several possibilities. The tumour—if that's what it is—could remain quiescent—or at least, it might not progress faster than her other diseases.

C: It could develop locally—it could ulcerate and fungate.

F: I've seen that. It's painful, ugly and smelly—very distressing for the patient. I wouldn't want that!

C: Or it could spread to other parts of her body—bones, brain, liver etc.

D: That sounds awful! You *have* to remove it! You can't just leave it to grow!

A: You can't do anything unless you know what it is. You have to establish the diagnosis. I think you have to 'recommend' a biopsy first up.

PK: All right. In fact, I did that. I arranged a fine-needle biopsy, where you suck a few cells up into a syringe and look at them through the microscope. It was unmistakeable: she had an aggressive carcinoma. What now?

B: I think you should raise with her the question of dying.

E: I disagree. She hasn't brought it up. You can't introduce it yourself. You can't say 'I know that you wanted to die once. Well, there's a good opportunity now!'

PK: It's true that in none of the time that I knew her did she ever say to me explicitly 'I want to die'. As I said before, she came close. On one occasion, when she seemed a bit depressed, she was contemplating the end of her life. She said, quoting, I think, from Shakespeare, 'It's silliness to live when to live is torment; we have a prescription to die when death is our physician'. I waited for her to go on, but she said no more, and the subject never came up again.

F: What happened? What did you recommend?

PK: Well, I basically did what C suggested. Because of the possibility of local spread and the pain and discomfort associated with that, I told her that I thought we should remove it and she readily agreed. The operation was conducted without a general anaesthetic and was uneventful. Pathology confirmed an aggressive cancer. She was also put on hormone therapy.

A: How did the wound heal?

PK: It healed OK. She continued to attend outpatients and to live with her sister. I really don't know how they managed, but they did.

One day, not long after the operation, she was clearly unwell and she complained that her cough was worse than usual and productive of thick, green sputum. On examination, she had a fever, but in view of her underlying chest disease it was very difficult to tell for certain whether there was any acute infection; nonetheless, clinically, I felt that there was evidence that she had pneumonia. What should I do?

G: Here we go again! I can't take any more of this! *(Mockingly)* 'What should I do?' All you need to do is ask her! She's a grown woman. She knows what she wants. Just give her the facts and let her decide for herself. The trouble with doctors is that they can't believe that their clients are autonomous human beings. It's all just a power trip!

(G gets up and leaves noisily)

PK: *(After a pause)* I think I must have said something wrong! Perhaps we should go on ...

F: Perhaps you could say something like 'I think you have pneumonia. This is an infection of the lungs. If we give you antibiotics it'd probably get better. What do you want to do?'

PK: Then, knowing her, Miss T would reply 'What do you recommend? My field's English literature, not medicine!'

B: Then you'd have to discuss the implications of the various alternatives.

PK: Well what are they? If she has pneumonia, she may well die ...

E: I don't think she really wants to die. She's never said to you directly that she wants to die. She's just gone through an operation to remove a breast cancer. She always takes her medications. That's not the behaviour of someone who wants to die …

B: Maybe she just doesn't want to suffer, as she said.

E: Let me finish! The only evidence that we have that she ever wanted to die was second-hand from her GP. She's gone though an awful lot since then. Who knows—maybe her life is richer and more satisfying than it's ever been before?

D: I agree with that. If she wanted to kill herself she could have done it herself months ago. She's intelligent enough. She could have taken all her pills at once or she could have found out what else she could do.

B: Would she need to come into hospital for antibiotic therapy?

PK: That would be one way of doing it—and the most effective. Alternatively, she could be given a course of oral antibiotics to take at home, with the option of a hospital admission later if desired.

B: Let's do that! If she doesn't want to take them she doesn't have to.

PK: Thanks for that—in fact, that's exactly what we did. We gave her oral antibiotics and the infection cleared. It has to be said, of course, that the clinical assessment was difficult and it is hard to say exactly what was going on. Anyway, she got better.

It was about two months later that the final, tragic chapter began. It was late at night. I was off duty at the time. Apparently, Miss T's sister came into her bedroom to ask if she wanted some Milo before going to sleep and found her on the floor, having a fit. She called an ambulance which took her straight to hospital.

She was seen in the Emergency Department by the intern and the registrar on duty and was noted to be in 'status epilepticus' (that means she was having constant fits). For some reason (without any reference to the treating doctors), she was immediately sent upstairs for a CT scan and then to the ward. The scan showed unequivocally that she had several large masses in her brain—almost certainly due to secondary spread of the breast cancer. She was given an intravenous drip, a nasogastric tube (that is, a tube through her nose extending down to her stomach) and anticonvulsant medications were commenced. *(Some groans and gasps are heard)*

When I saw her the next morning her condition was essentially as I've described. She was lying in bed with intravenous and nasogastric tubes. She was drifting in and out of consciousness with frequent, barely clinical fits. From time to time, she'd recognise me—enough at least to allow her to squeeze my hand in recognition—but she was unable to talk and certainly couldn't have a conversation.

What should we do now?

B: Let her die. Let her die. Now is the time to let her die!

D: But how? Would you kill her? Would you really, actually do it?

E: Is she in pain?

PK: There's no evidence that she's experiencing physical pain.

B: She's probably suffering psychological pain though. You could still give her enough morphine to kill her.

PK: Morphine in sufficient doses would kill her. However, opiates also have the property of reducing the fitting threshold, so that they might actually exacerbate the tendency to fit.

F: Perhaps you could stop all her drugs. What would happen if you did that?

PK: It's always difficult to predict with certainty. Her main drugs are to control cardiac failure. It's possible that her lungs would fill up with fluid.

D: That's terribly distressing. You can't let her drown.

PK: I am interested to know what people think. Should we stop any or all of her treatment?

A: I'd stop the heart drugs and treat her symptomatically if she becomes distressed.

PK: What about her anticonvulsant medication?

A: No. Of course you'd continue that. Convulsing would be extremely upsetting for her.

PK: What about her intravenous drip and the nasogastric tube?

A: I can't see any reason for an IV. In my unit we can almost always manage without an IV. We'd usually maintain a fine-bore nasogastric for giving drugs and fluids if necessary.

PK: Well what about that question? Should she be given food and fluids?

E: By law, she has to have 'reasonable provision of food and water'. You're not allowed to starve someone to death.

D: I've heard that it's very painful to die of dehydration.

A: That's not necessarily so. Anyway, if you need to, you can either give water through the tube or saline subcutaneously from time to time. We do that all the time.

C: I'd give fluids but not food.

B: That's illogical. If you're going to feed her you should do so properly. If you want her to die you should do the job quickly!

C: But what would you do? Would you kill her? I couldn't do that. I could stop giving her drugs and maybe not even feed her, but I couldn't kill her.

F: Can she say anything now? Can you ask her what she wants?

PK: No, unfortunately. It's definitely too late. There's no question that she's unable to give a coherent response to any question now. Signs of recognition—a squeeze of the hand, a weak smile—are all she is capable of. I should add that there was no advance directive or Enduring Power of Attorney, although I'm not sure that they would have made any difference.

E: It's not necessary anyway. We've had plenty of opportunities to find out from her what she wants. And in any case, what someone says under great duress can't be accepted.

PK: Our time's nearly up so we'd better settle it. Who thinks that we should feed her—that is, give her food? ... Only one person. Who thinks that we should give her water or fluids? ... Most.

Well, I'll tell you what happened. We removed the drip and kept the nasogastric tube, mainly to give her the anticonvulsants. We stopped the medications for her heart failure as suggested. We didn't give regular fluids: that was partly because her sister and niece spent a lot of time offering food and drink to her. In fact, the two of them maintained a vigil beside her bed, giving her spoonfuls of soup whenever she'd take it. It was extremely moving: they were there almost all the time—certainly, every time I came to see her, one of them was there.

Time passed—about two months, I think. Virtually nothing changed. She continued to drift in and out of consciousness and to have multiple, small fits. Her sister and her niece remained at her side, giving the spoonfuls of soup. At the end of that time she was skin and bones.

Then one day, her niece came up to me. She was very upset.

She said: 'This is just terrible! It can't go on. It's the worst of all possible worlds. It represents everything that my aunt never wanted. It's hell for her and it's hell for us!

'Do something!'

What are you going to do now?

Epilogue

In daily life, ethical issues are everywhere. We make frequent and continuous decisions about the small details of even the most mundane of our interactions. Typically, we assume a limited number of large-scale principles and we take into account regional codes of behaviour. However, the substantive contents of our face-to-face relationships are not set primarily by such principles or codes. Rather, they are negotiated in the courses of these relationships as they emerge out of our shared lifeworlds of social and cultural experience.

When we engage another person in almost any interchange, we embark on a process of mutual exploration that may lead to uncharted, unknown territory. If he or she is not an intimate acquaintance but someone I have come across in everyday life or my professional work, the experiences we have shared may be limited. Nonetheless, this does not diminish the fact that we are, from the outset, irrevocably bound to each other. We engage in dialogues and share experiences as we negotiate our way—not always without misadventure—through potentially explosive fields of conflicting values. We call on whatever resources are available to us: we advance ideas and arguments; we watch for, and try to accommodate, reactions; we call up past experiences and previous conversations. We may draw others into our relationship; we reflect on our interactions and then discuss them; we may even discuss our discussions. We reach an outcome, sometimes conclusive and satisfying, often partial, desultory and incomplete.

It does not always work smoothly, and often we encounter obstructions that prove insurmountable, as many of the stories in this book attest. For example, I may be perplexed about the seemingly irrational refusal of a patient such as Maria to engage in treatment of proven benefit for breast cancer in place of untested complementary medicines; I may struggle to understand the world of someone struggling with advancing illness and the burdens of a ruined childhood, as in the case of Elizabeth; or I may watch aghast as I witness the inexorable decline of a young woman like Jo, encumbered not only with the sad fact of her obesity but also with the cruel responses of an unsympathetic society. These difficulties, however, only emphasise the deep complexity and richness of everyday ethical discourse.

When I enter an ethical interaction—with Maria, Elizabeth, Jo or anyone else—our lives intersect and become intertwined. Together, we launch into a journey that leads into the unknown. At the end of the process we are both changed irrevocably. The practical dialogues that drive my daily life forward start from the inexorable fact of this enmeshment with others. Indeed, relationships with others come even before my sense of my own identity, before my own subjectivity. In contrast to commonly held assumptions, the latter actually arises from the former. My uniqueness lies precisely in my irreducible responsibility for others, a responsibility that I cannot evade and that I would not want to evade. This responsibility is mine alone: it establishes who I am and how I am differentiated as a free and autonomous human being.

Our contact with others is not primarily through ideas and concepts. We are connected both through language and through our shared corporeal presence in the world. This is especially relevant to medicine, of which the general currency is the physical experience of illness and disease. Our shared language enables us to share physical experiences, and at the same time our common, embodied world opens up new fields of meaning to which we have joint access. Words and carnal experience are themselves inexorably intertwined. On the one hand, our embodied experiences underlie the possibility of language. On the other, words can 'pick up and amplify the sonorities' latent in the things; they can 'resonate through the body and help it re-establish its inner rhythms and melodies'.[1]

Through language, we make and pursue our contact with the world of things and with other people. These other people appear as specificities or singularities within our fields of speech and language, and our mutual contact arises from an abrasion between our discrepant discourses. Our dialogues are therefore never seamless or straightforward. They are not processes of translation; they do not entail the realisation of pre-existing meanings; they are not the result of the application of a tool according to a formal procedure or a fixed algorithm. They cannot be separated from the acts of speaking themselves or from gestures that are often obscure and opaque[2], and which lead to the open and unpredictable creation of new meaning. They constitute an experiment and, as in all experiments, their outcomes cannot be predicted.

It is often pointed out that the unavoidable responsibility for the other that is the premise of my personal and social identity is also the grounding moment of love.[3] In love, an 'I' establishes a responsibility for a 'You' and in so doing accepts the other's radical otherness as unique. In this sense, all ethical contact is based on the presupposition of love. This is not to minimise the complexity and difficulty of ethical interactions, or that communication is usually imperfect, or that protagonists may occupy widely varying value positions, assumptions, philosophical dispositions and religious beliefs, in part because of the diversity of culture, in part because of the irreducible specificity of personal experiences, of love, pain, suffering and death. However, it does emphasise the equally important fact that, as difficult as ethical dialogues can be, the sharing of meaning can never be fully obstructed.

No matter how profound the differences are between us, we can always establish some kind of contact: it is always possible to make some sense, to share some degree of understanding. As the examples discussed in this book illustrate, communication can occur in the most difficult of circumstances through the deployment of a wide variety of expressive resources, through intuitive and unspoken connections that draw on broader cultural knowledge and embodied experiences, and through the creative use of language, including ambiguity and silence. The technics of ethical communication are complex and multifaceted. What is common to them, however, is that they commence with the suspension of narrow sets of rules about the production of truth or the identification of ethical validity and that they provide an opening to the fashioning of novel forms of meaning. When I face someone I do not understand—when I try to fathom the pain of Rebecca's traumatic history, when I try to understand Maria's apparent irrational rejection of the Western medicine that might save her life, when I attempt to interpret Miss T's conflicting messages—I seek a way to break through the curtain of unintelligibility. To achieve this, I have to suspend my own biases, to find a way to make contact on a different level, to listen in a different vein. I have to try to imagine, to re-create within myself, what she is getting at. As I listen to her talking, I try out images and possible meanings to see if they are plausible or carry compelling force. Rather than relying on a demand for causal explanations, I construct in my mind systems of categories of functional principles or qualities. My task is to identify common ground, a place where we can come together as individuals in the understanding of our mutual and diverse experiences. I open myself, carefully and deliberately, to a suggestiveness and an allusiveness from which the process of dialogue can progress.

In their work, scientists seek precision, univocality and the elimination of divergent shades of meaning. In ethical discourse and clinical communication, however, what is often required is the deliberate expansion of the range and scope of possible meanings and the preservation of uncertainty and ambiguity. When we encounter the implacability of otherness, its opacity and perverseness, when we sense that we are reaching the margins of sense, when, for example, Elizabeth is negotiating the limits of her own understanding and insight, when Jo expresses her despair as her options close off, we call on the expressive power at the edges of language. We rely not just on the words themselves, on their exact meanings. We call up the resources of ambiguity, of metaphor, of irony, or of the many other tropes available to help us to move forward to new territory. We become, literally, the poets of our lives, in the smallest, most everyday matters.[4]

In ethical dialogue we keep future possibilities open, however remote they may be; that is, we seek to maintain hope.

The construction of the future from within the present as an open array of potential events is always dependent on the ability to imagine possibilities that go beyond the certainties of the everyday, on utterances left unfinished, on strange metaphors, on silences. Similarly, ethical dialogues occur not only through formal processes of mapping across theoretical structures, but also by the exact opposite: through the location and mobilisation of the gaps in language, of the spaces in which meaning is not fixed, in which words gesture towards things, ideas, emotions and experiences, the rents in the flowing fabric of meaning. By allowing us to move within the shadow world at the boundaries of sense, these dialogues enable us to fashion ideas and ways of understanding that have never before acquired recognisable shape. Here we find weapons for conquering new territory, for driving beyond the conventional limits to the silent territory just outside what has hitherto been said or experienced.

These experiences or utterances cannot be separated from the concrete settings in which they arise. They are always rooted in a social and historical reality and in flesh-and-blood experience.[5] They are always subject to the absolute and irreducible specificity, and the infinite variety, of the shared lifeworlds that are their ground and their precondition. The connections that are established in the often troubled course of the ethical interchange are not the result of the application of formal tools or methods; they are not outcomes generated by formal, logical deductions. They flow out of the complected, embodied contact we make with others, out of the menacing but irresistible meeting of gazes across the unfathomable abyss of otherness.[6] The shared meanings of the ethical relationship arise out of the constant proximity of the other to us. Ethics, speech and face-to-face contact are not the outcome of a solitary or impersonal exercise of thought. They are part of a shared adventure of creation, discovery and sometimes difficult struggle.

One does not have to go to exotic places, seek out extreme circumstances or look for fundamental innovations in science, technology or culture to encounter the edges of experience and meaning. In the grey, commonplace continuum of the everyday, there is already heroism, joy, tragedy, suffering, honour, trust, loyalty, betrayal, altruistic caring and ruthless egoism. The lives and deaths described in this book were and are the lives and deaths of flesh-and-blood men and women. They express the richness of the fluid and tragic experiments of love and death, often partial, inchoate and incomplete, but always inexhaustible.

Notes
1. A Lingis, *The First Person Singular* (Evanston, North-western University Press, 2007), p. 62.
2. E Levinas, *Philosophical Essays* (The Hague, Martinus Nijhoff, 1990), p. 115.
3. ibid., p. 133.
4. F Nietzsche, *The Gay Science*, tr. Walter Kaufman (Toronto, Vintage Books, 1974), pp. 239–40.
5. F Nietzsche, *Thus Spake Zarathustra* (New York, Modern Library, 1937), pp. 198–9.
6. G Deleuze, *Essays, Critical and Clinical* (Minneapolis, University of Minnesota Press, 1997), p. 166.

Index

abjection, 241–2
abstract universalism, 9–10
Abu Ghraib, 202
Adorno, Theodor, 142
Aeschylus, 160
Agamben, G., 132, 204
alterity, 77, 82, 89–91, 93, 95–7, 109–10, 127, 129, 131, 134–7, 220, 235
anguish, 148–50
animal experimentation, 47–70
animal liberation movement, 48–70
animals, 52–4, 64–5
anthropocentrism, 57, 70
Apel, Karl-Otto, 35–6
archive, 132–3, 180, 189, 204
Arendt, Hannah, 130
Ariès, P., 166
Aristotelian ethics, 3, 8 *see also* neo-Aristotelian theories
Aristotle, 52
art, 13–14
Augustine, Saint, 143
Auschwitz, 126
autonomy, 20–1, 24, 41, 107, 110, 114

Bacon, Francis, 56, 165
Bakhtin, Mikhail, 84–5, 96, 129, 146
Barker, Francis, 86
Barthes, Roland, 186–7
Bataille, George, 222
Baudrillard, J., 220
Bauman, Zygmunt, 108
beauty, 13–14
Being and Time (Heidegger), 148
beneficence, 20
Berger, John, 87
Bernard, Claude, 37
Berrigan, Daniel, 234
Beslan, 141
bioethical discourse, 24, 67–8
bioethics: abstracted, 22, 25; criticisms, 8–10, 23–5; definition, 4, 33–4; industry, 21; limits to debate, 24–5; major schools, 8
bodies: disabled, 229–30; doctors', 74, 88; gender, 94–6; grotesque, 85, 240–1; lived experience, 80–2, 92, 110–11, 115, 128, 228–30, 239, 241–2; meanings, 73–87, 95–7, 111, 115, 128, 228, 230–4, 239–43; sick, 76–7, 80, 82, 96 *see also* obesity
Bordo, Susan, 231
Borges, Jorge Luis, 182, 216
Bosnia-Herzegovina, 141

Butler, Judith, 76, 79, 95

cancer: breast, 101, 159, 168, 254–8; ovarian, 106
caress, 88–9
Cassell, Eric, 32
childbirth, 30–1
clinical interactions, 16, 25–42, 77, 82, 90–2, 103, 108–10, 124, 129, 131, 134–6, 144, 254–60 *see also* physical examination
communication, 35–6, 40, 55, 67–70, 131, 267–9
competence, 20
Conrad, Joseph, 203
consequentialism, 51–2
crisis, 62–3
Cruelty to Animals Act [UK], 50
culture: cultural bias, 23; nature, 59–60, 65–7, 69
cyborgs, 219

d'Alembert, Jean le Rond, 56
de Waelhens, A., 86
death, 157–74, 216–17
Deleuze, Giles, 152, 182, 211–12
deontological ethics, 8, 53
Derrida, Jacques, 187
Descartes, René, 56, 111, 113
Diderot, Denis, 56–8
Diprose, Rosalyn, 114
discourse ethics, 12, 35
discourses, 13, 78, 84, 86–8, 91, 94, 97–8, 103–4, 116–17, 125, 128–9, 137
disruption, 77, 80–2, 92, 109–10, 112–13
doctors: archive keepers, 132–3, 180, 204; bodies, 74, 88; as witnesses, 130, 132–3, 163, 180, 203–4
Dostoyevsky, F., 160
Douglas, Mary, 76, 241
duty, 9

eating, 234–8
ecology, 51, 59–64
embodiment, 37

empathy, 131, 162
Enlightenment, The, 7–8, 52, 56–8, 68, 126, 128, 160, 165, 240
environment, 51, 59–64
epistemology, 4, 61, 126
eros, 89
eroticism, 89–90
'ethical life,' 9–10
ethics: Aristotelian, 3, 8; definitions, 55–9, 109–10, 116; deontological, 8, 53; discourse, 12, 24; evaluative, 9; global, 15–17, 116; Kantian, 8, 9, 26, 36; local, 15–17, 116; medical, 21–6; normative, 8–11, 15, 36, 91; postmodernism, 14–15; regional, 15–16, 116; utilitarian, 8 *see also* bioethics; microethics
Ethics (Spinoza), 152
Euripides, 139, 199
euthanasia, 171–3, 248–55, 261–4
everyday life, 102, 143–4, 269
evil, 139–54
existentialism, 13, 37, 90, 106, 112

Faust, 139, 185
feminism, 94–5
Foucault, Michel, 35, 37, 78–9, 83, 95, 132
Freud, Sigmund, 77, 86, 109, 221

Galen, 49
Galilei, Galileo, 7, 56
Gandhi, Mahatma, 234
gender, 73, 94–6
good, 17, 55, 91, 97, 143, 145, 147–8, 152–3
grief, 196–7, 221–2
Guantanamo Bay, 202
Gulag, 141
gynaecology, 83

Habermas, Jürgen, 10–12, 15, 35–6
Hamlet, 165, 182, 188
Heart of Darkness (Conrad), 203
Hecabe, 139, 199–200, 208
Hegel, Georg Wilhelm Friedrich, 8–10, 52

Heidegger, Martin, 8, 148–9, 161, 168, 183
Helvetius, 7, 57
heteroglossia, 96, 109
Hiroshima, 141
HIV, 193
Holocaust, 141–2
humanity, 13
Hume, David, 58
Husserl, E., 11, 14–15, 183, 187

identity, 108–9
Illich, Ivan, 165–6
illness, 92, 96
Iraq, 202
Irigaray, Luce, 94

Job, Book of, 149–50

Kant, Immanuel, 3, 7–11, 26, 58, 143, 146–7
Kapsalis, Terri, 83
Kierkegaard, S., 8, 160
knowledge, 13
Kosovo, 141
Kristeva, Julia, 241

La Mettre, 7
language games, 35, 39–40
Le Besco, Katherine, 232
Leder, Drew, 112
Levi, Primo, 204
Levinas, Emmanuel, 78, 82, 88, 148–50, 160, 183, 200, 219, 235–7
liberation, 7, 13, 57
lifeworld, 11, 40, 88, 90–1, 107, 109, 116, 145, 147, 234
Lingis, Alphonso, 130, 146–7
linguistics, 69, 125–7
Lockerbie, 141
love, 78, 267

Macbeth, 214
MacIntyre, Alasdair, 12, 58
Managayam, Dr, 193, 204, 208
Marx, Karl, 8
materialism, 58

meaning, 153–4
medical ethics, 21–6
'medical gaze,' 37, 104
Mei Lay, 141
menopause, 80–1, 101–18, 123–4
Merleau-Ponty, Maurice, 75, 77, 111–12, 135, 160, 232
microethics, 4–6; decision-making, 144–8; definition, 16–17, 33–4, 116, 136; domain, 26–34
modernity, 8, 12–14, 126
moral space, 107–9, 115
morality: Enlightenment, 7–8; goodness, 17; Hegelian, 9; Kantian, 9; reason, 68
Munich, 141

narratives, 179–89; 'grand narrative,' 13
nature, 51, 59–64, 67, 69
Nemo, Philippe, 149
neo-Aristotelian theories, 10–12
Nietzsche, Friedrich, 8, 95, 104–5, 109, 113, 118, 152, 185
non-maleficence, 20

obesity, 226–43
objectification, 83–4
Omagh County, 141
On the Genealogy of Morals (Nietzsche), 95

pain, 54, 72–3, 76, 92, 96, 112, 133, 196–9; animals, 47, 52–3
palliative care, 157–8, 164, 167, 169–72
Parmenides, 78
pathology, 74
Pellegrino, Edmund, 5
phenomenology, 4, 8, 183
Phenomenology of Perception, The (Merleau-Ponty), 75
philosophy, 8–12, 23, 56–7
physical examination, 26–7, 75, 82, 87–90
plague, 226, 231, 242
Popenoe, Rebecca, 231

Port Arthur, 141
positivism, 4
'post-structuralist' theories, 4
postmodernism: art, 14; definition, 13; ethics, 14–15; identity, 109
power, 78, 84, 89, 93, 95
proletariat, 13
psychoanalysis, 86–7

Rabelais, François, 96
reason, 7–9, 13, 58, 68
reductionism, 4, 93, 112, 114
resistance, 92–3
Ricoeur, Paul, 148
Rilke, R.M., 128, 137
Rousseau, Jean-Jacques, 52
Royal Society, 50
Rwanda, 141, 202

Sands, Bobby, 234
Saunders, Cicely, 167
science, 4, 55–9, 66–70, 96
self, 76–7, 83, 96, 126, 129
September 11, 2001, 202
sexuality, 74–80, 92–5, 97 *see also* bodies
SIEV X, 202
Signs (Merleau-Ponty), 75
Sittlichkeit, 10
Society for the Prevention of Cruelty to Animals, 49
sociobiology, 4
sociology, 6
Spinoza, Benedict de, 152
Srebrenica, 141, 192, 202
structuralism, 4
subjectivity, 12, 77–8, 127, 266
suffering, 73, 80, 82, 130, 149–50, 162–3, 194, 198–200, 202–5, 208, 249; animal, 52–3, 66
suffragettes, 234

superstes, 132
Sydenham, Thomas, 37
Symbolism of Evil, The (Ricoeur), 148

Taylor, Charles, 12
temporality, 161, 178–89
testis, 132
testosterone, 92–4
Toombs, Kay, 229
touch, 27–8, 87–90
Touraine, Alain, 109
Toussaint, François-Vincent, 68
trust, 28, 32, 134
truth, 13, 55, 78, 96, 127
Twilight of the Idols (Nietzsche), 185

universal pragmatics, 35
universalism, 9–10, 36
utilitarian ethics, 8
utilitarianism, 3, 7, 58

validity, 55
values, 14, 38–9, 69
Vietnam, 141
virtue, 12
voluptuousity, 89, 95

War and Peace (Tolstoy), 169
War on Terror, 202
Weber, Max, 14
witness, 130, 132–3, 162–3, 180, 203–4
Wittgenstein, L., 35
womankind, 13
Women of Troy, The (Euripides), 199

Young, Katherine, 74–5, 83

Zaner, Richard, 76
Zarathustra, 145
Zizek, Slavoj, 220

www.ingramcontent.com/pod-product-compliance
Lightning Source LLC
Chambersburg PA
CBHW052014070526
44584CB00016B/1744